THE
UNHEALTHY
TRUTH

THE
UNHEALTHY
TRUTH

How Our Food Is Making Us Sick—
and What We Can Do About It

ROBYN O'BRIEN
WITH RACHEL KRANZ

Broadway Books
New York

Published in the United States by Broadway Books, an imprint of
The Crown Publishing Group, a division of Random House, Inc., New York.
www.broadwaybooks.com

BROADWAY BOOKS and its logo, a letter B bisected on the diagonal, are trademarks of
Random House, Inc.

Library of Congress Cataloging-in-Publication Data
O'Brien, Robyn.
The unhealthy truth : how our food is making us sick and what we
can do about it / Robyn O'Brien with Rachel Kranz. — 1st ed.
p. cm.
Includes bibliographical references.
1. Food allergy in children. I. Kranz, Rachel. II. Title.
RJ386.5.O27 2009
618.92'975—dc22
2008054788

ISBN 978-0-7679-3071-0

PRINTED IN THE UNITED STATES OF AMERICA

1 3 5 7 9 10 8 6 4 2

First Edition

To my husband, my greatest blessing

———————————————

"The truth is incontrovertible.
Malice may attack it, ignorance may deride it,
but in the end; there it is."

—WINSTON CHURCHILL

CONTENTS

FOREWORD

The landscape of children's health has changed. No longer can we assume that our children will have a healthy childhood—certainly not in the face of the current epidemics of autism, ADHD, asthma and allergies, childhood cancers, childhood obesity, and diabetes. In fact, autism, ADHD, asthma and allergies, or the 4-A disorders, as I termed them in my recent book, *Healing the New Childhood Epidemics: Autism, ADHD, Asthma and Allergies,* have all increased dramatically in the last two decades. Approximately 30 million children—more than one-third of our kids—are affected by one of these four new childhood epidemics. This is not something we can just accept. This begs explanation.

We have witnessed a meteoric rise in the incidence of autism—at least 1,500% in the last two-plus decades. You cannot meet anyone these days who has not felt the reach of this epidemic, whether they have a child affected by autism or have a friend, business associate, or family member with an affected child. Autism has entered every walk of life, every profession, and every socioeconomic group. The statistics speak for themselves: in the United States, one in every 150 children is affected by autism. The numbers are even more staggering in New Jersey, where one in 94 children and one in 60 boys is affected. Some have tried to attribute this spike in incidence to better diagnosis. But although there has been expansion of the autism spectrum to include some more highly functional individuals, such as those with Asperger's syndrome, this does not explain the epidemic. A study by the MIND Institute in California in 2002 confirmed this fact as well. As I frequently say to parents, therapists, teachers, clinicians, and researchers alike, if that is the case, show me all of the thirty-year-old autistics. They're just not there. We are in the midst of a relatively new epidemic.

One in eleven children struggles with asthma, and one in four is affected by allergies. The incidence of allergy has increased significantly over the past two decades, and allergy to peanuts has more than doubled from 1997 to 2002. We have seen peanut butter banned from schools across the nation due to the number of children for whom contact with and in some cases even the smell of peanut butter may cause a deadly anaphylactic episode. The same disturbing trend holds true in the rise of childhood obesity and childhood onset of type II diabetes. There is something very troubling out there that is affecting our kids. We have all heard of the canary in the coal mine—the sensitive bird miners sent ahead of them to test the atmosphere. If the bird lived, they knew there was enough oxygen, but if it died, they knew they could go no farther. Sadly, our children have become those canaries, and those with lower thresholds for the toxicants that pervade our environment are being unmasked more and more.

My practice has seen thousands of children from around the country and the world who are struggling with these new epidemics, but we are not alone in witnessing these disturbing trends. Pediatricians across this country and around the world are seeing more of these children, and these physicians can tell you that the problems we see now simply did not exist two decades ago. These epidemics our children face are new, and we must find a way to reverse them.

There is a growing body of evidence that supports the belief that the increased incidence of these childhood disorders arises from a genetic predisposition coupled with environmental triggers or insults. Environmental insults to which our children are increasingly being exposed include common chemicals (such as PCBs, flame retardants, plasticizers, and pesticides), heavy metals (including mercury, lead, arsenic, cadmium, and aluminum), countless types of food additives, and an ever-increasing number of genetically modified foods. These environmental toxicants can increase oxidative stress (from extremely reactive molecules that damage cell membranes and other cellular structures), wreaking havoc on cellular function at all levels. Changes caused by oxidative stress can also lead to chronic inflammation, which may be a common underlying mechanism in many of the childhood disorders our children are experiencing. Thankfully, we are learning new ways to remediate oxidative stress through the use of dietary and supplemental antioxidants, such as fruits and vegetables; vitamins A, C, E, and carotenoids; the minerals selenium and zinc; herbs such as green tea, pycnogenol, and quercetin; and nutraceuticals such as coenzyme Q-10. Some of these antioxidant nutrients (including green tea, pycnogenol, and curcumin) also have anti-inflammatory properties, as does one of the most important natural anti-inflammatories: omega-3 essential fatty acids. As these epidemics continue and more of our children are affected, more research emerges to support this point of view. Also, increasing numbers of physicians and researchers are lending their support and expertise, shedding light on the factors contributing to these devastating disorders.

Robyn O'Brien's compelling examination of the effects that recent changes in our food supply are having on our kids cannot be ignored. Genetically modifying foods leads to the possibility of changing protein structures, whereby they are recognized as foreign to our immune systems. The immune system then attacks these foreign substances, but unfortunately may also overreact and attack the body's own cells, violating its primary credo, which is differentiating between self and non-self. This attack on self, initiated by these "foreign proteins," then leads to all types of autoimmune disorders and dysfunction.

Through comprehensive integrative treatment approaches, we have been able to help more and more children. Though our ability to help greater numbers of these affected children is gratifying from a therapeutic perspective, it is not enough. Prevention is the key, and in this regard, everyone needs to play a role—not only clinicians, physicians, researchers, and parents but also government and corporations. It always has been the parents who have been so important, raising their voices about the epidemics affecting their children and driving the quest for answers. The mothers and fathers I see every day are the most determined people I have ever met, refusing to accept the "gloom and doom" they have been fed about their child's condition and doggedly pursuing answers even when they are told there are none. We must reduce the toxic exposures to our children. The course of genetic conditions is difficult to significantly alter, but thankfully, there are no such things as genetic epidemics. Environmentally induced disorders connote more malleability, and the possibility for real change.

We must move beyond the treatment realm, which is where I live in terms of my caring for these children, and additionally focus on the realm of prevention. This is where the voice of a mother such as Robyn, with multiple kids affected by these disorders, plays such a crucial role. She is an inspiration to mothers around the world, showing that you don't have to sit back and watch the health of your children decline—you can take an active role. Founding AllergyKids, creating a Web site and a forum on the Internet for open communication, has helped Robyn to empower parents to enact changes in our society. She has alerted people to the dangers of our toxic environment, including our food and the adverse effects it has on our children, and this has placed her in the forefront of the movement for change. Bucking the powers that be in an "Erin Brockovich" way has made her simultaneously loved and admired by some and disliked by others, depending on their perspective and position. She has emerged as a true American hero and a beacon of light for our kids, for beyond treatment of affected children, prevention of these disorders in the next generation of kids is paramount. It can't be said too strongly: this effort must not be limited to physicians, researchers, and parents, but rather must also include government and our corporate structure to bring about truly significant change. To reduce our children's exposures to environmental toxins, it will take a vision and mission of truth, acknowledgment of contributing factors, and, most important, a change in policies and procedures. We must cooperate at every level to make our environment safer and less toxic for our children, and this is Robyn's passion and her life's work. It is what must be done. Our children deserve no less.

Kenneth A. Bock, MD, FAAFP, FACN, CNS
Author of *Healing the New Childhood Epidemics: Autism, ADHD, Asthma and Allergies;* www.rhinebeckhealth.com

It seemed like an ordinary day. My oldest three gobbled up breakfast with their usual appetite. The baby was fussy, maybe tired, so I put her down for a nap. The next thing I knew, her face looked like an angry, swollen, red tomato and I had plunged into the midst of a childhood epidemic I barely even knew existed.

Now, I grew up in Houston, where I ate my share of Twinkies and po' boys growing up, since my sweet mother's main concern was feeding *her* four children without busting the food budget. Until this day, I had been completely clueless about food allergies, which is what my pediatrician diagnosed when she saw Tory that afternoon.

Luckily, a megadose of antihistamine was enough to relieve my daughter's symptoms. But my own journey was just beginning. After all, I was a mother, and my baby had just gotten sick—really sick, in response to some very ordinary food that I had given her. I couldn't stand the idea that there was nothing I could do about it. I *had* to find answers.

And so, after putting Tory to bed and reassuring the other kids and talking to my husband and doing all the other normal, crazy-busy chores that are part of raising a family of four, I started looking. It was a search that began that January day and hasn't ended yet. But the more answers I thought I had found, the more questions emerged. What had changed in our food to make it suddenly so toxic to our children? How had PB&J and a carton of milk become loaded weapons in the lunchroom? When had food—one of the most immediate, personal ways I knew to sustain my kids—become so friggin' *dangerous*?

The more I learned, the more overwhelming the problem came to seem. I was stunned at how prevalent food allergies had become in the last ten years—at least one out of every seventeen children under the age of three suffers from them, more than double the number a decade ago. I was even more shocked to realize how little information there was about this rapidly growing condition and to discover corporations with vested interests in the issue were funding—and skewing—what little research was being done. It floored me to learn that the system that was supposed to guarantee us and our families safe, healthy food had broken down a long time ago and had been replaced by a revolving door between the FDA and the very corporations that it's supposed to regulate.

In the course of my journey, I've learned a lot. I've discovered that one out of every three U.S. kids currently suffers from allergies, asthma, ADHD, or autism and that the number of children with peanut allergies actually *doubled* between 1997 and 2002. I'd love to give you more recent statistics about what may well be America's fastest-growing health problem, but since there's so little government or private industry funding for that kind of research, those statistics just don't exist—that's another thing I've learned.

I've also found out that genetically engineered products are in virtually every bite of processed food we eat. I've learned that no one, not even the most ardent defenders of genetic engineering, can say for sure how these altered foods might affect us or our kids. I've also unearthed a pile of studies on the effects of additives, artificial coloring, and aspartame, studies that have prompted governments around the world to remove these chemicals from their food—studies that most of us have never heard of. Although moms and dads in England, Europe, and even South Africa are assured by their governments that their children won't be exposed to such dyes and additives as tartrazine (a.k.a. Yellow 5) and the risks these chemicals pose, we U.S. parents are barely even told about the problem.

Overall, I've learned that the food we're eating—even the food we thought might be the healthiest—is often dangerous to our health. One of the worst symptoms of the problem is the growing allergy epidemic, but the problem is hardly limited to people with allergies. All of us—and especially our children—are in potential danger from genetically engineered soy, corn, rice, and potatoes; hormone-laden milk; and the high-fructose corn syrup, synthetic colors, and artificial sweeteners that seem ubiquitous.

Full disclosure: I was raised on capitalism and the *Wall Street Journal,* and from the time I was a kid, I believed in our system and its leaders. Finding out about the dangers lurking in my daughter's plate of eggs was bad enough. Discovering the corporate corruption, government cover-ups, and outright greed that have broken our system was enough to break my heart. I didn't like learning that part of the story, not one bit. But I do want to share it with you, because I believe that once we understand the problem, we can work together to solve it.

Maybe that's the most important thing I've learned: that no matter how frightening, or overwhelming, or just plain confusing this food issue seems to be, there *are* things we can do about it, just as mothers in Europe, Australia, Asia, and other developed countries around the world already have. We can make our voices heard, just as those moms have, in our schools, on TV, to our government, in our kids' lunchroom. We can make big changes or little ones, recognizing that as one of us moves just one tiny step forward, we all move forward together. We can talk to other parents and work with them. And we can clean up our kitchens, and our kids' diets—in ways that are cheap enough, easy enough, and delicious enough for even the busiest parents and the most resistant kids.

Small Changes, Great Rewards

Over the past two and a half years, lots of folks have asked me how I kept going all this time. Learning about the dangers in our food supply was so overwhelming—why didn't I just give up? Coping with my kids'

allergies was so scary and time-consuming—why didn't I just concentrate on them and leave the big picture alone? Switching from our old diet to our new, healthy one seemed so impossible—why didn't I just give in?

Well, in some ways, the questions contain their own answers. I had four kids, and my Mama Bear instincts were engaged. I *had* to protect every one of them. And once I knew that everybody else's kids were also at risk, I couldn't just ignore that danger. So no matter how hairy things got—and sometimes they got pretty hairy—giving up was not an option.

But also—and this is the most important part—every time I took a positive step, I got a reward. Maybe it was something big, like seeing my son Colin's eczema clear up or hearing his lifelong cough go away after we cut milk and dairy products out of his diet. Maybe it was something small, like watching John smile when he crunched a carrot or knowing I'd given Tory a breakfast that was safe for her to eat. Maybe it came from outside, like all the e-mails I got from parents who'd been fighting this battle for years and were so glad to know they weren't alone. Maybe it came from within, just that warm feeling you get when you know you've done something good for your family.

One of the biggest rewards in this whole process has been the sense of being part of something larger than myself. I'm far from the only mom who's concerned about the safety of our food supply, and I *know* that every other mom and dad out there wants to do right by their kids. Feeling how much we can accomplish when we all work together has been incredibly inspiring for me. Knowing that we're all in it together has really helped.

Once, when I passed those bright-blue boxes of Kraft mac 'n' cheese in the grocery store, I was filled with despair, guilt, and maybe some anger, too. Why were *our* kids being dosed with the chemicals that gave the powder its bright-orange color when the kids in England weren't? Why were we being sold products laden with genetically altered ingredients, without even the courtesy of a label warning us what our kids were being exposed to? Moms in Europe and Great Britain didn't have to agonize over which boxes to buy: corporations there had voluntarily

removed many of the worst chemicals and slapped a "genetically altered ingredients" label on the box.

Now, when I pass those boxes, I feel hopeful. Parents in Europe, in Russia, in Australia, in the Philippines, and in South Africa *have* managed to make the corporations listen. They've gotten their governments to take action. They've succeeded in protecting their children. That means we can do the same. Hope, I've discovered, is an incredibly galvanizing force.

Not that it's been an easy journey. When I started down this road two and a half years ago, my biggest obstacle wasn't always in the grocery, or the boardroom, or the FDA. It was that little voice in my head saying, "You're no scientist. You're no doctor. You can't even cook. Who in the world is going to listen to *you*?"

It's hard to ignore that little voice, let alone talk back to it. It's especially hard if your parents, or your siblings, or your neighbors, or your pediatrician is adding to the clamor, insisting that you don't know enough, aren't smart enough, have no business sharing your opinion.

But I've come to realize that we have to find a way to speak out anyway, little voice or no. In my case, I draw confidence from remembering that I'm a former equities analyst who earned a Fulbright grant and spent years researching multibillion-dollar deals, which has put me in an excellent position to understand the economics—and the corporate politics—behind our current food crisis. And while I'm not a scientist, I've spent years talking and sharing e-mails with some of the top researchers and physicians in the field. So even though I'm not a scientist, I can share those resources with you.

You may have similar skills to draw on, or you may have different ones. Maybe you're a teacher who knows how to put complex ideas into simple language, so everyone can understand. Maybe you're a paralegal who can explain the twists and turns of the legal system to your neighbors. Maybe you're a busy parent who—whether you wanted to or not—has become a skilled multitasker.

Whoever you are, whatever you do, I promise you: You *can* be an expert on your own family's health. You *can* make a difference, both at home and in the world. All you need is enough courage to take the first step. You can figure out the next one later. And as each of us takes a step, even the tiniest step, we all move forward together. Arm in arm. Kids in tow!

So if you're out there trying to do right by your family, if you care about your own health, or if you're concerned about the health of future generations, then you're the person I wrote this book for. We *can* turn this thing around and provide healthy, nutritious, delicious food for our families. We *can* get our government to listen to us, the way the governments in Europe and Australia and Japan have responded to *their* citizens' concerns. We *can* make it easier to be a parent—because honestly, folks, it *shouldn't* be so hard!

1

BABY STEPS

I've never been one to do things halfway. As the oldest of four children, I got every single one of those "first-born" traits—you know, the type A, compulsively driven type? When I was in business school, I was relentless about always doing the best job that could possibly be done. It wasn't as much to win that A from the toughest professors as it was to set the bar as high as I could: to see what I might accomplish and to keep life interesting.

Along the way, I fell hook, line, and sinker for my husband, Jeff, whose unconditional love never wavered in the face of my passion and perfectionism. I mean, the man must have patience in a bottle! He kept me going through business school and then through my career as an equity analyst in Houston. And when I launched into full-time motherhood, he continued to support that same type A mentality as we knocked out four kids in five years.

It was an extraordinary adventure, but I won't pretend it was easy, especially at mealtimes. If you've ever cooked for even one child, you know what I mean. When they come downstairs on Saturday morning, you want to be ready for anything—tears, songs, fights, whatever. You don't even know whether your kids are going to be dressed or immobilized, unable to make a move until you find them the blue football shirt with the yellow sleeves that they wore yesterday.

Sure, I wanted to give them healthy food in some form or fashion. But Martha Stewart didn't live in my house! As a cook who had been known to burn pancakes, I was less interested in culinary excellence than in just covering the basics.

So on the morning of January 21, 2006, that's what I tried to do. Trying to appease four hungry children, I gave Tory, my youngest, some banana while handing each of the older three a tube of bright-blue yogurt. Then I threw the frozen waffles into the toaster, slung the syrup on the table, and scrambled up some eggs (which I had also been known to burn).

Five-year-old Lexy, my oldest, was quiet that morning, off in her own world as she dreamily ate the yellow mass I quickly dumped on her plate. Four-year-old Colin was cranky but busy sucking down that blue yogurt, so at least he wasn't fighting with his three-year-old brother, John, who kept up his usual running stream of commentary and questions as he and Colin gobbled up their meal. As I passed Tory, smiling placidly in her high chair, I realized that she'd never yet tasted eggs and remembered that my pediatrician had suggested I start introducing her to new foods, one at a time. So on one of my many trips between the toaster, the frying pan, and the kitchen table, I slipped a few spoonfuls of eggs onto the tray of her high chair.

Out of the corner of my eye, I noticed that Tory wasn't exactly eating her eggs. It was more like she was playing with them, the way babies do. She was also becoming fussy, so half an hour later, as the other kids trooped off to play in the family room, I put her down for her morning nap and put her leftover eggs onto a piece of toast for my husband.

What I really wanted to do next was sit down and read the paper, but with a pile of dirty dishes, that wasn't an option. And of course, the last thing I was inclined to do was check on a sleeping child, because, as every parent knows, naps are gifts! Maybe when Lexy was first born I made a few extra trips into her bedroom, but by the time Tory came along, I had learned to let sleeping children lie until I heard that unmistakable wake-up call or perhaps a cry of distress, usually the result of a decision by John to torment his baby sister.

So I don't know what made me go upstairs that morning a few minutes after I put Tory down. Maybe it was mother's intuition, one of the many "Mama Moments" I had learned to recognize and prize as my surest guide in those first years of motherhood. Whatever the reason, I poked my head into Tory's room—and was stunned. My baby's face was bloated and puffy and red. She wasn't crying or even fussing, but her face was so swollen that her eyes were shut.

I snatched her out of the crib and ran down to the family room. I'm sure my panic spooked my other three, who looked at me with baffled eyes. "What did you guys *do*?" I burst out, trying not to shout. "What did you put on Tory's face?" But they just stood there, giving me those blank little-kid stares. The ones that let you see straight down into their little souls—those deeply honest stares when you *know* your kids are telling the truth.

That's when I really got scared.

Trying to regain my calm, I made my way to the phone and called my pediatrician, Tory cradled in my arms. "Robyn," the doctor told me, "it sounds like an allergic reaction. What did you feed the children for breakfast?"

When I told her—milk, waffles, eggs—it appeared to confirm her suspicion. I later learned that milk, wheat, and eggs are three of the top eight allergens. Although virtually any food can provoke an allergic reaction in somebody, some 90 percent of all food allergies are triggered by the proteins in eight foods: eggs, cow's milk, wheat, soy, fish, shellfish, peanuts, and tree nuts, such as walnuts, almonds, and Brazil nuts.

You have to be kidding me, I thought when the doctor gave me the news. Wheat, eggs, and dairy were everyday staples in our house. How had such ordinary foods—the foods of my childhood—become so dangerous?

"Just bring her in," the doctor told me, so I left the other kids with Jeff and drove Tory to the hospital in town. My little sweet pea, with her hugely swollen face and little slits for eyes—she looked as though she'd been in a fistfight. I couldn't believe that something I'd fed her could have hurt her so badly.

After talking with me further, Tory's doctor decided that those scrambled eggs were probably the culprit. Being a baby, Tory only had two teeth, so she hadn't had any of the waffles, and of course, she was too young for milk. Today was the first time she'd tried eggs, though.

No, said the doctor, that couldn't be right. A child's first allergic reaction to a food is almost always the result of a second, third, or even later exposure to that food's protein.

"But that makes no sense," I insisted. "Tory has never eaten eggs before. Today *was* the first time."

The doctor reminded me that Tory had just had the flu vaccine a few months earlier. Since the vaccine was grown in eggs, today's breakfast was actually Tory's second exposure.

"Does this mean Tory can't get vaccines either? And that she can't eat anything that's made with eggs—cake, cookies, waffles? Will she outgrow this? Is there anything I can do?" It was terrifying to think that such brief, minor contact with something that seemed so healthy could produce such a dramatic reaction.

The doctor shrugged and my mind raced. *Great,* I thought, *my daughter can't eat, she can't get her vaccines. What is going to happen to this kid?* My heart sank as the doctor explained that even when a child tests positive for allergies, it's often not clear how severe they are or in what circumstances they might be triggered. I wanted her to tell me what I could do to fix my kid. But she couldn't.

Later I would learn there were two diametrically opposed schools of thought on childhood allergies. One group of experts maintains that you should expose your child to small amounts of the foods to which she is allergic, hoping that contact will permit her to outgrow the allergy. A second group insists that you have to keep your child away from the offending food, hoping that *lack* of contact will permit her to outgrow the allergy. There's no real medical consensus on which approach is better, although the proponents of each approach are sure that the other only makes the problem worse. If they had set out purposely to drive a mother crazy, they couldn't have done a better job.

Even though she wasn't absolutely sure what had caused Tory's reaction, the doctor gave Tory an antihistamine, which to my enormous relief began to work almost immediately. I strapped my daughter into her car seat and drove home. "Since when did an *egg* become so dangerous to someone in our family?" I asked myself. "How insane is that?"

Leggo That Egg, Kids!

The first order of business, after getting Tory settled back into her crib (between the antihistamine and missing her nap, she was pretty tired), was to talk to the rest of my kids. I knew it had scared them to see their sister so sick and me so distraught, and I wanted to reassure them as soon as I could.

But, I must admit, I also wanted to terrify them. Not really, of course, but it crossed my mind. One thing I had grasped from that trip to the doctor: Tory was allergic to something, probably eggs, but maybe other stuff, too. So if John was "a good sharer" and handed her his Eggo waffle, or if Lexy lovingly held a glass of milk to her sister's lips, as she had with both her younger brothers, could they be endangering Tory's life? For all I knew as of that morning, yeah, they easily could be. How could I make my kids aware of that, especially John, who was only three? How could they learn not to endanger Tory without coming to view her either as a ticking time bomb or as the most annoying burden?

Well, the first step was talking about it. "Hey, gang," I said when I had gathered them around the kitchen table, "you know how Tory was so sick this morning, right?"

John looked up at me, his eyes round. He *must* have been spooked, because you usually couldn't get this busy three-year-old to stand still for so long.

Four-year-old Colin shrugged, but I knew he was paying attention. Five-year-old Lexy, my mother's helper, nodded, her eyes wide, too.

"She's okay now," I reassured them. "But what we learned from this is that there are some foods that you guys can eat that Tory can't. And so we're gonna have to figure out a way to protect Tory in our house and make sure that we don't accidentally give her the wrong foods." I paused, looking down at their serious, upturned faces. "Do you understand?"

Again, Colin shrugged. John's eyes had already wandered off somewhere else, and I remembered the parenting book that had said that if you wanted a toddler to remember anything, you literally had to say it fifty times. Lexy, the only one who really seemed old enough to take it all in, said, "What do you want us to do, Mommy? How can we help Tory?"

"Okay, guys. Here's the new rule. *Never give Tory anything to eat.* Nothing at all. Get it? Mommy is *the only one* who can give food to Tory. So if you want to give her something, *ask Mommy first.*"

Well, as you can imagine, this wasn't the easiest rule for my kids to remember. I'm not sure John ever did get the concept. Colin never gave any sign of understanding, but he never gave Tory anything, either. Lexy, who even at five was such a tuned-in, compassionate child, understood that her baby sister, Tory, couldn't monitor her own food intake and that Mommy really couldn't be everywhere at once. So she took it upon herself to be my little reporter.

"Mommy," she'd say, running over to where I was frying up eggs or working at the computer or maybe running the vacuum cleaner over the hall carpet, "John just gave Tory a Cheerio!" Or "Mommy! John just gave Tory a piece of his banana!"

"John," I'd say, wondering how to get this confusing new rule through my little boy's head, "don't you remember what we said about Mommy being the only one to give Tory food?"

John would look up at me with his angelic, mischievous smile, and I'd think, *How the hell is he supposed to understand this? He only just turned three!* He'd seen me give Tory a few Cheerios or a slice of banana, so he knew it was food she liked. He hadn't seen anything bad happen when I gave it to her. So how in the world could he understand why he wasn't supposed to hand his little sister a bite of perfectly harmless food?

The worst part of the whole thing was that I knew it wasn't just going to be John. Eventually, I'd have to leave Tory with a sitter, or drop her off at the church nursery, or take her to preschool, or even let her go to a friend's birthday party. I couldn't just wrap her in cotton wool and keep her safely at my side, much as I sometimes wished I could. I couldn't tattoo "Food allergies—NO EGGS" on her forehead, either, much as I fantasized about doing *that*. (It wouldn't have helped with John anyway—he couldn't read!)

Meanwhile, above and beyond the problem of keeping Tory away from eggs, which we were pretty sure had set off the first attack, was the general lack of knowledge. There was that first three weeks between taking her to the pediatrician and our desperately awaited appointment with a busy pediatric allergist. And then there was that frustrating time *after* the allergist's appointment, because he really didn't have any answers either, even though I had a whole long list of questions.

Was Tory allergic to anything other than eggs? Probably not—but she might develop more allergies, or she might already be allergic to something, or several things. Given her age, she was too young to test properly because her immune system wasn't fully developed. We wouldn't know the whole story until she was at least three.

Was Tory at risk for any other conditions? Maybe asthma. Asthma and allergies often showed up hand in hand. But there was no way to test for it and no medical protocol for prevention (though I still believe our superhealthy diet did in fact keep her from getting asthma).

Was there anything I could do to make the allergies go away or to prevent her from getting new ones? It was hard to say, really. They just didn't know.

Why were so many kids suddenly developing these scary food allergies? Was this a new epidemic? Well, the experts couldn't really agree on that one. Anyway, the specialist assured me, that wasn't really my problem. *My job was keeping Tory safe.* Only he couldn't really tell me how to do that, either. (I did eventually find *some* answers to those questions, which I'll share in chapters 2 and 3.)

I began to search the Internet, looking for answers the doctors couldn't give me. I set up my laptop on the dining room table—adjacent to our eat-in kitchen, where the family meals were held—and began to hunt. My old training as an equities research analyst kicked in.

Allergies: The New Childhood Epidemic

Much of what I initially learned about allergies turned out to be incomplete. For example, the official statistic holds that allergies affect some 7 million Americans, including about 6 percent of children below the age of three. That information comes courtesy of U.S. Food and Drug Administration Deputy Commissioner Lester M. Crawford, DVM, PhD, speaking before the Consumer Federation of America on April 22, 2002.

You may be wondering why I'm quoting a statistic that's more than six years old. And that's part of the problem: in the last six years, there has been virtually no research to give us definitive statistics on the number of kids with food allergies. If, by the time this book comes out, your kids are under seven, then chances are that the data you've been given is older than your kids are.

Still, most experts agree that the incidence of allergies is "skyrocketing," to use Dr. Crawford's word. Similar testimony comes from Robert Wood, MD, pediatric allergist at Johns Hopkins Children's Center and author of *Food Allergies for Dummies*. "Over the last 20 years . . . the prevalence of food allergy appears to have risen sharply," writes Dr. Wood.

Or consider the candid comments of Dr. Jacqueline Pongracic, head of the allergy department at Children's Memorial Hospital in Chicago.

She's quoted in a 2006 article published online in *Pediatric Basics,* written by another of our nation's most prestigious physicians and research scientists, A. Wesley Burks, MD, professor and chief of the Division of Pediatric Allergy and Immunology at Duke University Medical Center. Dr. Pongracic explains: "I've been treating children in the field of allergy immunology for 15 years, and in recent years I've really seen the rates of food allergy skyrocket. Where in the past it only represented a small proportion of my practice, now more than half of the children I care for have a food allergy."

One of the few hard figures we do have comes from a study published in the *Journal of Allergy and Clinical Immunology* in late 2003. This article cited a statistic that I was to hear—and quote—many, many times in the coming months: that the prevalence of peanut allergies among children had doubled between 1997 and 2002, increasing from 0.4 percent to 0.8 percent.

Are allergies really increasing that quickly? I thought when I ran across that figure on that first afternoon of Tory's illness, back in 2006. *Let's do the math.* If peanut allergies had doubled in that five-year period, that meant they'd gone up an average of 20 percent a year. Could that possibly be right?

I looked at the figures again. Yes, a 100 percent increase in five years meant a 20 percent annual increase. But if that was the case, wouldn't the numbers still be increasing? Why would the allergy rate have begun to jump in 1997 and then stopped suddenly in 2002? Just because the study had ended didn't mean the problem was solved.

And was the rate of increase still 20 percent per year? Had it slowed down, or might it even be accelerating? After all, the experts seemed to agree that food and other allergies were "skyrocketing." Indeed, wrote Dr. Burks, "Estimates have been that from 6–8% of children under 4 years old have food allergies, but some experts believe the percentage is growing."

Clearly, the problem was getting worse. But since no comprehensive studies were being done, no one knew exactly how much worse.

The little research that's been done since my first foray into the subject confirms that allergy rates continue to skyrocket. As a matter of fact, one of the only food allergy studies conducted by the Centers for Disease Control (CDC) in the last eight years shows a 265 percent increase in the number of hospitalizations related to food allergies.

I've also learned that it's not just food allergies that are on the rise. According to a November 2007 article in *Newsweek,* hay fever—a.k.a. "seasonal allergic rhinitis" or sensitivity to the pollen from trees, ragweed, or grass—has shot up since 1996. The article cites the National Center for Health Statistics (NCHS) as saying that in the past ten years, the number of children with seasonal allergies has jumped from 6 percent to just under 9 percent. I don't even need my calculator for that one: that's a 50 percent increase! And in the opinion of Dr. Marc Rothenberg, director of allergy and immunology at Cincinnati Children's Hospital, "The severity of those allergies has also increased."

After years of playing the numbers as an equity analyst, such figures make my antennae go up. Why is this condition affecting more children? What's behind this sharp decline in what the experts call "the age of onset" for peanut allergies? What other allergies are appearing at earlier and earlier ages? And most important: What's causing this dramatic increase in allergic reactions, especially to food? Has something in the food changed?

Of course, some experts advise caution, suggesting that perhaps we *don't* have an allergy epidemic. Dr. Burks's 2006 article also quotes Dr. Scott Sicherer of the Mount Sinai School of Medicine: "There are no studies in this country looking at whether the rate of food allergies has increased over long periods of time."

When I read that quote, all I could think was, *Why the hell not?* Why *hadn't* a potentially life-threatening, skyrocketing epidemic—one that had threatened not only my child but millions of others—become a top research priority?

But on my first forays into research at my dining room table, I was ready to take the figures I read at face value. Although I now believe that the standard figures of "one in seventeen children" or "6 to 8 percent" are outdated and therefore far too low, when I first began to learn about this problem, all I could think was that my Tory was part of a nationwide epidemic—an epidemic I had barely heard of.

The Tip of the Iceberg

I now believe that food allergies are really just the tip of the iceberg. They don't just affect the children who have them—they're a warning sign from our kids' immune systems that something is wrong with our food supply. This toxic food supply has not only created an allergy epidemic, but also is linked to other types of health problems, such as asthma, autism, ADHD, and behavioral difficulties, as detailed in Dr. Kenneth A. Bock's internationally recognized book *Healing the New Childhood Epidemics.* Kenneth A. Bock, MD, FAAFP, FACN, and CNS, is the head of the Rhinebeck Health Center and has practiced medicine for the past twenty-five years. He's become a trusted colleague, has appeared on *Good Morning, America* with me, and was kind enough to write the foreword for this book.

You can certainly find many scientists who will pooh-pooh the connections that Dr. Bock asserts—scientists who will downplay the role of diet in these various conditions. But you can also find a great deal of scientific evidence to support it. To cite just one provocative example, a study in Great Britain discovered that many children with antisocial, disruptive, and/or criminal behaviors tested positive for food allergies. When the allergens were removed from their diets, their antisocial behavior declined significantly.

As I learned more about food allergies, I came to see our allergic kids as "canaries in the coal mine," warning us of problems that could affect the health of us all, whether we suffer from a specific allergy or not. But in order to grasp the big picture, we first need to understand the allergy epidemic. So here's a quick look at the ABCs of food allergies.

Food Allergies and Inflammation: When the Cure Is Worse Than the Disease

An allergy is basically an overreaction by your immune system to a protein that it perceives as a threat—for example, the proteins in particular types of food, the dust mite protein, or pollen. For people without allergies, these proteins are harmless. But if you've got an allergy, your immune system sees these proteins as dangerous invaders.

To drive the invader out, your immune system mobilizes all its resources: mucus, to flush out the intruder; vomiting, to force it out; diarrhea, to expel it quickly. Such conditions may make you feel sick, but they're actually evidence of your body's attempts to get well.

A key aspect of the immune response is known as *inflammation,* characterized by one or more of four classic symptoms: redness, heat, swelling, and pain. Inflammation doesn't occur only in allergic reactions; it flares up whenever your body feels threatened, in response to a bruise, cut, bacteria, or virus as well as to otherwise harmless pollen, dust, or food. Scientists now believe that much of our immune systems is found in our digestive tracts, where many of these inflammatory reactions occur in the form of stomachaches, cramping, nausea, bloating, and vomiting.

Ironically, the immune system's inflammatory reaction—meant to heal and protect the body—often causes more problems than the initial "invader." The eggs my daughter tasted that fateful January morning were dangerous to her not because they were intrinsically toxic but because of the inflammatory way her immune system responded: with redness, swelling, hives, and fever. And if the swelling had included not only her face but her respiratory system, her allergic response might have caused her throat to swell, threatening her ability to breathe and perhaps even killing her.

When I first read that information, I had to pause and take a breath. *How am I supposed to protect my daughter from her own body?*

Still, I had to marvel at all the different ways our bodies have discovered to protect and heal themselves, even if some of those ways create problems of their own. It's as though the body had developed its own "Special Ops" emergency-response team, with high-speed vehicles, the latest in automatic weaponry, and skilled marksmen ready to shoot down any invader.

Put that team up against a real killer, like cancer or a deadly virus, and you've got a body ready to fight its way back to health. But set that team against a misunderstood invader—such as the protein from a peanut or an egg—and you can imagine the traffic accidents, broken windows, and wounded bystanders left in its wake. That's the irony of an allergic reaction: the body's attempt to protect itself can actually cause severe harm.

Let's take the most basic inflammatory reaction: redness, warmth, swelling, and pain. Every one of these responses is the result of the body's attempt to heal itself.

First, blood rushes to the affected part of the body, desperately trying to bring protective white blood cells to the battle zone. All that blood makes the area turn *red* and feel *warm*.

Then, the white blood cells release their protective chemicals, meant to heal. But these chemicals may leak into surrounding tissues, causing them to *swell*. And the whole process—again, meant to heal—often stimulates the nerves, causing *pain* (or sometimes itching).

Depending on what is causing the inflammatory reaction, symptoms may also combine for a kind of flu-like effect, including fever, chills, fatigue, loss of energy, headache, loss of appetite, muscle and joint stiffness.

If you're already familiar with food allergies, you'll realize that many of the reactions I just listed are not to be found on the traditional list of food allergy symptoms. So here's where things get slippery. Although some of these symptoms are associated with food allergies, they're also associated with another type of food-based reaction most commonly known as *food sensitivity.*

Food sensitivity is another type of reaction that draws on a related but slightly different aspect of the immune system than food allergies do. Food sensitivities also produce slightly different symptoms, though there is also some overlap (see box, p. 20). Many doctors insist on an ironclad distinction between "food allergies" and "food sensitivity." But many other physicians and scientists, especially those more recently educated in the importance of diet and nutrition, see a significant link between the two conditions. Still other physicians refer to "immediate" and "delayed" food allergies.

Even though doctors don't always agree on how to classify these two types of reactions, a growing number see the two responses as aspects of the same problem. In both cases, the immune system is overreacting to an apparently harmless substance.

Common Symptoms of Food Allergy: Immediate Reactions

- rash or hives
- nausea
- stomach pain
- diarrhea
- itchy skin
- eczema
- shortness of breath
- chest pain
- swelling of the airways to the lungs
- anaphylaxis

Common Symptoms of Food Sensitivity: Delayed Reactions

- fatigue
- gastrointestinal problems, including bloating and gas
- itchy skin and skin rashes like eczema
- brain fog
- muscle or joint aches
- headache
- sleeplessness and sleep disorders
- chronic rhinitis (runny nose), congestion, and postnasal drip

Asthma and Allergies: When the Immune System Overreacts

There's a third type of inflammatory immune-system overreaction: asthma. Just as allergic people overreact to apparently harmless food, people with asthma overreact to apparently harmless substances or conditions—dust, pollen, cold air, mild exertion. In fact, many scientists see these responses as related, giving rise to such organizations as the American Academy of Allergy, Asthma and Immunology and the Asthma and Allergy Foundation of America.

In an asthma attack, as in an allergic one, the body's attempt to drive out a perceived invader may be more dangerous than the invader itself. Sometimes, inflammation causes an asthmatic's lungs and throat to swell so much that they block the person's airways, with potentially deadly consequences.

People with food allergies also suffer from that symptom, known as *anaphylaxis*. As I learned about this frightening new word, I discovered that it was derived from the Greek words *ana,* meaning "throughout," and *phylaxis,* meaning "protection." So in anaphylaxis, when a foreign invader is introduced, the body seems to turn its protective mechanisms on itself. *My God,* I thought. *What if that happens to Tory?*

If you're like me, you're now wondering just how many people—and how many children—die of food allergies each year. But we'll have to wonder in vain, because even the Centers for Disease Control doesn't track the number of deaths caused by food allergies.

However, the CDC does track the number of deaths caused by asthma, which is responsible for a shocking four thousand U.S. deaths annually, or eleven deaths each day. And every day, according to the Asthma and Allergy Foundation of America, asthma causes 40,000 U.S. residents to miss school or work, 5,000 to visit the emergency room, and 1,000 to be admitted to the hospital. The foundation also reveals that "asthma and allergies strike 1 in 4 Americans or an estimated 60 million Americans."

Think about that for a minute. One-quarter of the people living in the United States has either asthma or allergies. What's causing our immune systems to overreact like this?

It gets worse, because, as with allergies, the rates of asthma are skyrocketing. According to Dr. Robert Wood in *Food Allergies for Dummies,* "Reliable asthma studies show at least a 100 percent increase in the prevalence of asthma (an allergy-related disease) over the last 30 years. . . . [E]xperts believe that similar mechanisms likely underlie the dramatic increases in all allergic diseases."

Clearly, *something* is causing our immune systems to overreact. People with food allergies overreact to food; people with asthma overreact to other stimuli. But what is knocking our immune systems out of whack, causing them to overreact at all?

I wouldn't learn the answers to these questions until I'd been asking them for several months—and I'll share what I found in chapter 2. But before we look at the *why,* we're not yet done with the *how.* How else do inflammatory reactions affect our bodies?

The Cancer Connection

One of the most powerful aspects of the allergy response is the body's release of *mast cells.* These immune-system warriors are also part of the Special Ops emergency-response team. And, like other members of the team, they can be extremely helpful, highly dangerous—or both.

Remember how allergies begin: An allergic person encounters a protein, and her body identifies it—rightly or wrongly—as a toxic invader. So her immune system manufactures molecules, known as immunoglobulin E (IgE) antibodies, which are specially designed to attack that protein the next time it shows up.

As they lie in wait, ready for the next attack, those IgE molecules attach themselves to mast cells. The next time* the allergic person encounters the allergen—the protein that triggers this whole defense—the mast cells rush to the affected area and spray it with powerful chemicals known as cytokines and histamines.

Those chemicals are intended to knock out the "toxic invader," which they may well do. But they also produce other symptoms, including a runny or stuffy nose, breathing difficulties, and all the other allergic symptoms we've come to know so well. That's why doctors prescribe *antihistamines,* to fight the effects of the histamines.

So when the body is facing real danger, mast cells help fight off the intruders and repair the damage. But they also cause dangers to the body itself, above and beyond the allergy symptoms. For example, an April 24, 2008, study published in the *New England Journal of Medicine,* linked mast cells with a possible increase in pancreatic cancer.

In fact, inflammation generally has been linked to a number of health problems. As we've seen, it's a central aspect of autoimmune reactions, including asthma and allergies, as well as rheumatoid arthritis and fibromyalgia, a disorder characterized by the presence of chronic widespread pain. Many doctors also believe inflammation contributes to other disorders, including obesity, diabetes, heart disease, and cancer.

Learning about this information in the abstract is upsetting enough. Researching it as part of an attempt to understand my daughter's illness was overwhelming and at times quite terrifying. But I think I've finally got a handle on it. So here's my best summary of what we're up against:

1. Allergies of all types are skyrocketing, to the point where we are now facing a genuine epidemic.
2. The CDC and other government agencies are failing to fund studies to calculate the number of children affected.

---

*Sometimes an allergic person won't react the *next* time she encounters an allergen, but will react the third time, the fourth time, or a few years later. That's what makes allergies so tricky—we never know when an allergic person might have a severe reaction. We might not even have known that she *was* allergic until she had the reaction.

3. Related conditions, such as asthma, are also on the rise, which most experts believe indicates a widespread environmental problem affecting our immune systems.

4. The potential dangers of these conditions go far beyond the immediate discomforts of runny noses and itchy skin. Because of the long-term dangers of allergy-induced inflammation, supposedly harmless allergic reactions may actually be creating long-term health problems for ourselves and our children, including obesity, diabetes, heart disease, and cancer.

The dramatic increase in the number of people with allergies should serve as a warning to all of us that something about food has changed. In the next chapter, I'll look more closely at the possible causes of the allergy epidemic and propose some answers to these troubling questions. First, though, I want to shed light on the relationship between *food allergies* and *food sensitivity.*

Food Allergies and Food Sensitivity: Our Immune System Overreacts Again

At first glance, the distinction between "allergies" and "sensitivity" may seem like a meaningless word game. But understanding the relationship between these two conditions is crucial to grasping the true nature of the allergy epidemic—and to seeing how even the supposedly healthy foods in our kitchens may be harmful to our health.

As we've seen, allergies are an overreaction of our immune system, a kind of exaggerated response to a perceived danger. When Tory came in contact with those eggs, for example, her immune system "recognized" the egg protein as dangerous, just as it would have seen the danger in the bacterium that causes pneumonia or the virus that causes mumps. In response, her immune system created special fighter proteins called antibodies designed to identify and neutralize the "egg invader."

As we've seen, these fighter proteins are known as immunoglobulin E, or IgE for short. When they're released into the bloodstream, their purpose is to seek and destroy the invader, which they do by creating one or more of the classic food allergy symptoms, such as the hives from which Tory suffered, or the diarrhea with which other children respond, or, in more extreme cases, the anaphylactic shock that can kill a child within minutes.

As I discovered with Tory, the classic IgE response occurs within minutes or even seconds because IgE proteins are some of the most aggressive antibodies we know. That immediate IgE response is the defining characteristic of an allergic reaction.

Food sensitivities start out in a similar way. If a "sensitive" child is exposed to a protein that his system perceives as a threat, he'll manufacture another type of fighter protein, known as immunoglobulin G, or IgG. Although IgE and IgG antibodies appear to play similar roles, they produce somewhat different—though often overlapping—symptoms.

A crucial difference between the two, though, is their reaction time. The less aggressive IgG antibodies typically produce a delayed response that might not appear for hours or even days after the child has consumed the offending food.

So even though food sensitivities and food allergies both produce painful, inflammatory, and potentially dangerous responses, this delayed reaction time has led many doctors to give food sensitivities second-class status. Partly that's because they don't present an immediate and obvious threat to children's lives: only the IgE proteins trigger anaphylactic shock, for example, and in that sense, only the IgE proteins can "kill" (though the IgG reaction can have serious long-term consequences). I also think that traditional doctors tend to downplay the importance of nutrition, frequently dismissing the idea that such symptoms as earache, eczema, crankiness, brain fog, and sleep problems might be related to a child's diet.

However, an article in *The Lancet,* Britain's most respected medical journal, casts another light on the subject. The article referred to doctors who use elimination diets—diets that begin with a very limited, "safe" array of food choices and then add potentially problematic foods back into the diet, one by one.

The reason for adopting an elimination diet is to identify which foods in your diet might be triggering symptoms like skin rashes, fatigue, or stomachache. Often, some foods affect us without our realizing it and we live with the symptoms, taking medicine to alleviate the suffering. But if you eliminate these foods from your diet, you may find that your symptoms disappear. What becomes even more interesting is that when you reintroduce the offending food, you may suddenly suffer drastic symptoms that make it clear that the food was indeed triggering one or more problems. An elimination diet can sometimes reveal with dramatic speed that a particular food you've always believed was harmless is actually causing such chronic symptoms as headache, digestive problems, and even more serious complaints. Masked by your daily diet and by the slowness of the food-sensitivity reaction, the offending food does its dirty work without you ever realizing that it is the culprit behind your—or your child's—disorders.

When you take a break from eating that problem food, however, and then add it back into your diet, you see how powerful its effects are and how responsible it may be for a seemingly unrelated problem. Foods that you thought were safe for you turn out to be highly problematic, indicating the presence of a previous undiagnosed food sensitivity. As a result, the authors of the *Lancet* article conclude that the prevalence of food sensitivity (referred to in the article as "food intolerance") has been seriously underestimated.

Certainly, food allergies are far more dramatic. Whenever you read about a kid who died within minutes of eating at a fast-food joint or after breathing in the peanut dust from a friend's candy wrapper, that's an IgE-mediated food allergy: they're fast, they can be deadly, and I'm thankful doctors want to give them the attention they deserve.

But I also think doctors should be looking at delayed reactions, too, the IgG-mediated responses to food sensitivities. Some doctors do look seriously at both. Most conventional doctors, though, tend to focus on IgE immediate reactions. I think there are lots of reasons why they should view the two types of reactions as part of a larger, single problem.

First, both reactions stem from the same cause: the immune system's overreaction to apparently harmless food. According to internationally acclaimed author and physician Kenneth Bock, MD, there's also quite a bit of overlap between IgE and IgG symptoms. Both can contribute to inflammatory responses in multiple body systems.

True, the delayed IgG reactions are less likely to cause hives and are more likely to produce a host of apparently vague symptoms, such as headache, brain fog, sleep problems, joint pain, fatigue, and muscle aches. But both the immediate and the delayed responses are immune system problems triggered by a supposedly harmless food protein.

Second, both types of responses are skyrocketing, suggesting that both are symptoms of the same larger problem. "Both categories have been exploding in the past twenty years," Dr. Bock told me recently. "There are all kinds of adverse reactions. . . . A significant percentage of people have *something*."

In my opinion, conventional doctors' tendency to separate IgE-mediated food allergies and IgG-mediated food sensitivities into two separate problems has the effect of minimizing the allergy epidemic. Remember, IgE allergies, IgG sensitivities, and asthma—three similar ways that our immune systems can overreact—are all on the rise. Doesn't that suggest that there's something out there—in our environment, in our food supply, *somewhere*—that's producing this sudden spate of over-reactions? When we look at those three conditions together, we can see that there's a big problem out there, and it's growing. In chapter 2, we'll take a closer look at *why*.

Detecting "Hidden" Food Allergies in Our Kids

Meanwhile, we parents need to look at our kids and determine whether the supposedly ordinary childhood conditions that send us running to the pediatrician's office are actually the result of food allergies, food sensitivities, or, sometimes, both. I was astounded when I first learned that many common childhood ailments may result from diet, including chronic ear infections, coughs, runny noses, and headaches; eczema and itchy skin; and frequent sleepiness, listlessness, crankiness, or sickness.

If your child suffers from symptoms like these, perhaps her immune system is overreacting to the proteins in that apparently healthy glass of milk, or to the soy protein that's now added to almost every processed food, or to the high-fructose corn syrup that sweetens everything from sugar-free cereals to whole wheat bread. Research out of England also suggests that children may develop food sensitivities in response to "junk food," including the highly processed foods loaded with additives, fake colors, and artificial sweeteners. (I'll tell you more about that in chapter 6.)

So we need to realize that many apparently unrelated conditions in children—and, often, in adults as well—may have their roots in allergies, food sensitivities, or both. In fact, it's perfectly possible for someone to have an allergy *and* a sensitivity to the same food, with a host of symptoms that appear unrelated until you look at the person's diet. If your child seems to suffer unduly from the symptoms I've listed, you might want to look for a physician who can help you explore some dietary changes before looking into other treatments.

As the mother of four children who *all* turned out to have food allergies (not even food sensitivities, in our case), I only wish I had known how often seemingly routine, ordinary childhood illnesses are rooted in food. As I'll explain in chapter 6, I eventually discovered that my son Colin has a fairly severe allergy to dairy products, which kept him suffering for years with eczema, stomachache, headache, and chronic ear infections. I still cringe when I think of the way I smeared him with steroid-based creams, pumped him full of antibiotics, and put him under for ear-tube surgery when just taking milk out of his diet would have done the trick.

"If only I'd known then what I know now" is a common refrain among parents. Don't you often feel that you're just a couple of months behind the learning curve—that you've found out what you *really* need to know just a little too late to help your child?

Well, now you can benefit from *my* research. So here are the three things I wish *I'd* known three years ago! Maybe they'll be helpful to you:

1. *Even if your kids can't talk, their skin speaks volumes!* Did you know that the skin is a person's largest organ? I didn't—but wow, does that explain a lot. Even when your kid is too young to tell you how he feels or too used to her symptoms to identify them (when kids hurt all the time, they don't know they hurt), you can often read your child's condition in his or her skin.

Does your kid have eczema? Does he get rashes around the mouth, especially after he eats a certain food or swallows a certain beverage? Rashes around the knees, elbows, or armpits? Does he have "allergic shiners"—that is, dark circles under the eyes?

These are all inflammatory reactions, signs that the body is trying to rid itself of what it perceives as a toxic invader. In your child's case, that "toxic invader" might be an apparently harmless food, to which your kid is either allergic or "sensitive." Keeping that invader away from your kid may bring relief from symptoms—and it may clear up other problems, such as brain fog, crankiness, sleep problems, inattention, acne, and mood swings.

When I first realized that the skin was an organ too, it gave me a bit of a chill. *If that is what's going on* outside, I used to think, looking at Tory's welts or Colin's eczema, *what in the* world *is happening* inside? But since we can't see inside, let's at least give the outside a closer look!

2. *The toilet bowl has a lot to tell you.* Your kids' bowel movements, not to be too delicate here, also speak volumes. Before I realized that Colin had a food allergy, I never realized that runny poops are a sign that a person isn't properly digesting his food. And indeed, as we got the allergens out of my son's diet, his poops firmed up.

Understanding this little fact led to one of the grosser parts of our journey toward health. I had to tell my son, "Colin, when you do a poop, will you come tell me before you flush it?" *So* much fun! But worth it in the end, as my son's health improved and we could stop that endless stream of antibiotics—and the money that flowed straight out the door to the pediatrician's office!

3. *Chronic ear infections are often a sign of dairy allergies.* In our house, the slogan "Got Milk?" quickly morphed into "Got Eczema?" "Got Diarrhea?" "Got Ear Infections?" Sad but true, that ubiquitous white beverage has many ill effects for children who are allergic or sensitive to it.

So if your son or daughter seems to be complaining of frequent earaches, try substituting juice or water for the white stuff and see if that makes a difference. If your child also becomes livelier, more cheerful, and more attentive in school, you'll know you're *really* on to something.

Baby Steps

That first day after taking Tory to the doctor, all I kept thinking was "What has changed in our food that has made it so dangerous?" This question has led me to some unsettling answers and disturbing new questions, which I'll take up in the rest of this book. I have to admit, they were things that I didn't really want to know. But when I looked at my four little kids that day, I realized that the risk of *not knowing* far outweighed any fear of what I might find out.

Meanwhile, as I was searching for answers to my bigger questions, I was also trying to create new answers right there in our kitchen. One of my first reactions, when I understood that Tory's allergies were related to her immune system, was to think "immune system–cancer–danger!" My second reaction was, "Wow, a lot of people I know fight cancer by going on an all-organic, super-healthy diet. That makes sense—it sounds so *clean*. Okay, Tory's going organic!"

Now, I'm a bit embarrassed by how naïve that sounds. But I'm also relieved that I had that thought, however confused and unscientific. "Clean food" just seemed to make sense for my baby's challenged immune system. Even though I didn't understand the *real* reasons for going organic—the actual dangers that might be in our food supply and the link between those dangers and Tory's allergies—at least I understood that changing Tory's diet might help keep her healthy.

So my first step in our journey toward health was putting Tory on a diet of organic baby food. (When I use "organic" in this book, I mean "grown without any chemical pesticides or fertilizers and without genetic engineering.") Eventually, I let her have some Cheerios, banana, and some of the other foods that I discovered were safe for her to eat. But especially during those three weeks between our emergency and my appointment with the allergist, I didn't want to take any chances. Tory had safely eaten baby food before, so she could probably eat it now. And organic baby food seemed "cleaner" and more pure than regular, so organic it would be.

It's a sign of how uninterested I was in thinking about food that I made no changes whatsoever in any of the rest of our diets. Why should I? *We* didn't have food allergies! *We* didn't have special needs! Only Tory did— so Tory's needs would get met. The rest of us could continue as we always had.

I'd always dismissed people who paid all that extra money for organic food and made all that fuss about their diets—please! *I* wasn't like that and never would be. It was only that Tory had a special condition, that was all. A special condition that not even my doctor could tell me how to cope with. I had to do *something*. But I wasn't going to stop rolling my eyes.

Still, when I bought that first jar of organic baby food for Tory, I was really taking a baby step of my own, toward a whole new world of healthy eating and new understanding. And those first few baby steps would eventually lead me to some pretty remarkable places.

2

BECOMING THE ALLERGY DETECTIVE

It was a relief to get Tory home from the doctor that first day, but my relief was short-lived. Since my baby had three lively older siblings ages three through five, I knew that I couldn't completely control her food intake, however much I wanted to. I was desperate to protect her from her brothers and sister, especially from three-year-old John. But I could see after our first little talk that John remained oblivious, and so my desperation grew.

The more I thought about it, the more anxious I became. Sure, Tory was just a year old, so other than an occasional babysitter, Jeff and I were pretty much the only ones who fed her. But what would happen when she got even a little older? I had been totally clueless about allergies just a week ago, so how could I send her out into a world of adults and children who might be offering her food, at an age when she was barely able to say her name, let alone to explain that there were foods she couldn't eat? What if one day she didn't remember that she wasn't allowed to have eggs, or didn't realize that hidden eggs were lurking inside, say, an Eggo waffle or a slice of birthday cake?

I didn't want my daughter to grow up fearful, the need to explain her allergies foremost in her mind. But I hated the thought of her being so vulnerable. And the Mama Bear in me simply would not accept that there were limits to my ability to safeguard my child. There *had* to be some way to warn her and her siblings away from "danger foods," some way to eventually carry that message out to her preschool, the church nursery, her friends' birthday parties . . .

I wondered if there might be some kind of universal symbol that other parents used to protect their kids, something I could use to protect my daughter from her siblings. Once again, Mama Bear provided the impetus and Research Wonk provided the means as I jumped onto the computer, searching for ways that other parents had handled this problem. Obviously, I was hoping for a magic bullet, but a universal symbol would have to do.

Unfortunately, there wasn't one. No matter how much I searched, I couldn't find any hint of a sign or symbol used to indicate that a food might be dangerous to a kid who had allergies. There wasn't even any symbol for "allergies" in general—no equivalent of, say, the pink ribbon for breast cancer.

I had to wait three weeks for an appointment with the allergist, and that was just more inaction than I could bear. At least creating a warning sign was something I could *do,* some way I could at least *tell* myself that I was protecting my daughter. So I began to sketch my own.

Almost immediately, I thought of a stop sign, a symbol that would cue people to STOP before feeding Tory so they could find out what she could and couldn't eat. Wouldn't that be a good idea? We could put a stop-sign sticker on foods in our house that Tory couldn't eat, and that would help my other kids know what might be safe to give her. Or I could slap a sticker on a brown paper bag when I sent Tory to school with her lunch, to remind her classmates to stop and think before they offered her food. If I couldn't be there to talk for her, then maybe the stop sign could.

With a pile of scratch paper and a jar full of crayons, I eventually came up with a green stop sign bearing an exclamation point. The bright-green octagon seemed like an easy, kid-friendly way to get children to stop and pay attention, something that would grab their interest but wouldn't be scary or make Tory feel bad. I had grown up with fluorescent green "Mr. Yuck!" stickers denoting poisons under the kitchen sink, so the color seemed like something everybody could recognize and understand. It had been a roller-coaster of a day, but as I fell into bed that night, I somehow felt better. Finally, something I could *do* to protect Tory.

The next morning, when Jeff came in to breakfast, he thought the symbol was terrific. Then I shared with him a thought that had been slowly nudging its way into my brain.

"You know, Jeff, it's been unbelievably difficult finding information about allergies—there are several Web sites out there, sure, but they all seem to have the same three paragraphs, sometimes even word for word. It's driving me crazy. What if—"

I took a deep breath to give myself courage. After all, we had just had four kids in five years. Wasn't this sweet man due for a break?

"What if I started a Web site to provide free information about food allergies?"

In retrospect, I can't even remember how long we talked about this idea or how long it took me to develop a plan. I only knew that the idea seemed to take shape with dizzying speed. A few years earlier, I'd helped Jeff start his own financial services company, so I already knew how to register a business name and a domain name and to file the paperwork with the state. After a few days of research, I decided that my new Web site would be called AllergyKids.

As Jeff and I talked through the details, I realized once again what a remarkable man I had married. He had supported my compulsive devotion to business school and had encouraged me to save every dime I had earned as an equity analyst. Now he suggested that I take those savings and use them to launch AllergyKids.

I loved the idea of giving parents a quick and easy way to get the free information they so desperately needed. But Jeff and I could only fund this project for so long; then, somehow, the idea would have to be self-supporting. I was committed to providing free information to any parent who wanted it. But how could I make this operation self-funding?

My second idea dawned as I stared at the stop-sign symbol: I could make stickers. I couldn't be the only mom who wanted to label allergy-safe food for her kids. In fact, maybe we could sell other products that parents needed, like tags for kids' backpacks and special lunch boxes.

I conducted the first of what would be many online focus groups by sending out a quick e-mail query to a few trusted friends. Within a few hours, I'd gotten the "go for it" response I had been hoping for. Over the next few weeks, after hearing from a dad who hated having to carry his kids' allergy meds in his wife's cosmetic bag, we came up with a little medical case for carrying EpiPens, the single-dose injectors of epinephrine that many children used as an emergency treatment for an anaphylactic reaction. And for parents who were traveling with their kids, we designed a computerized wristband that could be used anytime, anywhere, to access their children's medical records. The project seemed to fill a real need, helping both Tory and the thousands of "allergy kids" who shared her condition.

But my biggest interest was in promoting the green stop sign as a universal allergy symbol. I hoped the symbol could maybe bring about a truce in what I'd come to think of as the "peanut-butter battle."

If you're a parent, you've probably seen it, too. The parents with allergic kids want to protect their children by banning certain foods from the lunchrooms. The parents of "regular" kids don't see why they and their children should have to suffer just because some children have special needs. I'd been firmly in the second camp, rolling my eyes at the allergy parents and mindful of the fact that two of my kids ate *only* peanut butter and jelly sandwiches. I sure wasn't interested in having "food fights" with my kids or in broadening my culinary repertoire.

But now my doctor had told me to protect Tory from a potential peanut allergy by not exposing her to peanuts in any form. Those PB&Js that Lexy and John adored now seemed like loaded weapons, pointing straight at Tory.

With the new battle lines drawn at my own kitchen table, I could finally see both sides. Of course the "food-allergy" parents were terrified that their kids might be offered peanut butter, egg salad, milk—foods that could make their children sick or even kill them. Of course the "non-allergy" parents were frustrated by the various restrictions imposed on their kids' diets or by learning to make new foods. Wasn't it hard enough packing lunches every day without accommodating *other* people's children?

Maybe my new symbol could help bring both groups together. Maybe it could enable non-allergy kids to bring in whatever lunches they wanted while the green stop sign on the allergy kids' lunch boxes reminded everyone to stop and think before they shared food. Maybe my new symbol could help educate children, teachers, and even parents, creating a safer, friendlier environment for everybody. If we could find a common solution, I thought, then we could all have our cake and eat it, too.

But I wasn't just thinking about parents and children. With my MBA background, I was also wondering how I could engage the business community. After all, in our society, it's the corporations who have the money. To create a national awareness of this problem, we would need to have them on our side. What incentive could I provide to engage them?

I had learned on the trading floor that corporations tend to pay attention and are a lot easier to engage if there is money to be made. Though some nonprofits do a fabulous job of fund-raising, I didn't want to compete with them—business was my area of expertise, not nonprofits. What if I designed a business model whose mission was to fund a cure for food allergies?

Inspired by the way Paul Newman had started Newman's Own to support environmental and other causes, I decided to operate AllergyKids along the same lines, with my own profits funding research and education on food allergies. I also thought that a for-profit model would engage the business community not just as donors but as partners, with forward-thinking food companies and grocery stores licensing my symbol and maybe even developing new allergy-safe food lines targeting this growing segment of the population.

As my idea took shape, I realized that plenty of businesses were already capitalizing on what I now saw as a—sadly—growing market. I'd heard of parents who had started allergen-free cupcake and cookie companies, and I would soon come to know women who had published children's books and cookbooks, or whose companies made EpiPens and similar products for allergic kids. I was happy to think that I, too, could help raise money for the cause, with every extra nickel going back to fund research and the spread of information.

Providing information was especially important to me, since the largest and most respected of the food-allergy nonprofits, the Food Allergy and Anaphylaxis Network (FAAN), wouldn't provide more than the most basic information until you paid its $75 membership fee. I joined, of course, and I respected the good work that FAAN was doing. But I didn't understand how they could insist that parents pay for information.

The way I saw it, if my kids were at risk, anybody's kids could be at risk. And if something could help my kids, maybe it could help other children, too. Weren't we all working for the same goal?

When I first broached the idea with Jeff in our kitchen, I had no idea where founding AllergyKids was going to lead me. But I guess I knew, even then, that there was no way I was going on this journey all by myself. Somehow, some way, a lot of other folks were going to be part of it.

Becoming "The Allergy Detective"

I'll be honest: one of the scariest experiences of my life was finding out that Tory had a food allergy. I understood—intellectually, at least—that what she had was probably not life-threatening. And when the allergist finally confirmed that she was allergic to eggs, I felt an enormous sense of relief. At least now I knew what to protect her from.

But along with the relief, I was terribly frightened. During that first visit, the specialist had also told me that Tory's allergic reaction meant that she was at an increased risk for other food allergies and maybe for asthma as well. As I listened to the confusing, contradictory advice that the allergist laid out for me, I felt as though my head was going to explode. Raising four kids was hard enough. Was I really up to these new demands?

Beneath the fear, of course, was guilt—an overflowing, super-sized portion of what I now think of as Mama Guilt, the feeling that perhaps without even realizing it, you've done something that has damaged the life of your child. That guilt had kicked in six months into motherhood, when Lexy, my oldest, got her first fever. Suddenly I realized that another human being was completely dependent on what I chose to do. How had I let her get sick? Had I fed her something that was bad for her? Let her teethe on something dirty? Taken her to the wrong park? Put her in the church nursery when other sick kids were there?

If you've got kids, you know exactly what I'm talking about, realizing that every choice you make could profoundly affect your child's life. Although it was tough to shake the feeling that I was somehow responsible for Tory's illness, a larger part of me kept wondering: *What is behind the new allergy epidemic?* That was the question that plagued me. And when I finally started finding answers, I've got to tell you, I wasn't too happy with them. It began to seem that this new epidemic was the sign of deeper problems with our health and our food supply—and, ultimately, with our political and economic system.

The Environmental Hypothesis

The first thing I discovered is that many experts have simply thrown up their hands in despair. In "Food Allergies for Dummies," for example, author and respected pediatric allergist Robert Wood, MD, admits that "No one really knows . . . what's causing this apparent sudden rise in food allergies."

There is some evidence that food allergies have a genetic basis. According to the Asthma and Allergy Foundation of America, if one parent has an allergy, his or her child has a one in three chance of also being allergic, while if two parents have allergies, their children's chance of being allergic are as high as 70 percent.

However, the children and parents don't necessarily share the same allergies. For example, a parent might have hay fever, while the child develops a peanut allergy. According to Dr. Andrew Saxon, chief of clinical immunology at UCLA, "The human race hasn't changed that much genetically in the last 200 years."

So if our genes haven't changed, then the epidemic must be caused by our environment. What has changed there?

One possibility is that such environmental pollutants as diesel exhaust and cigarette smoke are contributing to the rise of allergies. According to the research conducted by Saxon and his colleague David Diaz-Sanchez, environmental pollution is closely linked to the allergy epidemic.

Another possibility is suggested by Dr. Kenneth Bock. In his book *Healing the New Childhood Epidemics,* he argues that children are exposed to increasing levels of toxins, heavy metals, and pollutants. When I spoke with him, he added that the increased levels of environmental toxins are almost certainly throwing our immune systems out of balance.

As Dr. Bock explains it, our immune systems include powerful components known as T helper cells. I think of these T helper cells as the Terminator Team, including both the friendly, helpful "good cops" and the stern, get-the-job-done "tough cops."

T helper cell 1, or TH1, is the good cop. Only instead of helping little old ladies across the street, it focuses on the health of our other cells, protecting them against viruses, fungi, and cancer.

T helper cell 2, or TH2, is the tough cop, the one that gets angry and beats up on any substance that the body considers a toxic invader. As we saw in chapter 1, these toxic invaders include bacteria as well as otherwise harmless allergens, such as dust (in the case of asthma sufferers), pollen (for those with hay fever), and certain types of food (for people with food allergies).

In Dr. Bock's opinion, the surge in environmental pollution has led to a severe imbalance in our immune systems, skewing them too far in the direction of the "tough cop" TH2 function. Instead of accurately reading the potential dangers in the environment, these "skewed" immune systems are far too quick to overreact, just like a jumpy tough cop who pulls out his weapon and shoots at a backfiring car or a falling box.

"An allergic reaction is your body overreacting to something that it shouldn't react to," Dr. Bock explains. "These extra toxins create an immune environment that is more prone to that overreactivity." Or, as I saw it, too many tough cops on the beat, too much outrage and inflammation in the streets.

Although Dr. Bock's explanation of immune function is pretty standard, he's one of the few scientists to link the immune system to the allergy epidemic in that particular way. But he does go along with the most commonly offered explanation for the allergy epidemic, which is known—misleadingly, in my opinion—as the hygiene hypothesis.

Understanding the Hygiene Hypothesis, or "Is My House *Really* Too Clean?"

The hygiene hypothesis was first proposed by researcher David P. Strachan in a 1989 article published in the *British Medical Journal*. Since this was years before the food allergy epidemic, Strachan wasn't looking specifically at food allergies but rather at the common allergic conditions of hay fever and eczema. He noticed that these diseases were more common in smaller families than in big ones, even though you'd think it would be the opposite: the more kids per family, the more chances a child has to be exposed to an infection. Why, then, were the kids with fewer exposures getting sick more often?

Strachan thought that perhaps the exposure itself was helpful. The kids from the bigger families, he reasoned, were indeed exposed to more infections—and so had more chances to build up their immune systems.

Since 1989, scientists have used the hygiene hypothesis to explain why allergies became far more prevalent after industrialization, and why they're currently more common in industrialized countries than in rural ones. They claim that our kids simply aren't being exposed to enough dirt, animals, and good old-fashioned germs.

More recent research by Dr. Dennis Ownby of the Medical College of Georgia suggests that children who grow up with two or more cats or dogs are less likely to be allergic—not just to pet dander, but to other substances as well. This has led to speculation, again, that children "in the old days" who grew up closer to animals were somehow benefiting from the exposure.

In *Food Allergies for Dummies,* Dr. Wood adds that allergies are less common among children who grow up on farms, attend day care, and have many older siblings (though that last factor certainly didn't apply to Tory, the youngest child of four!). Again, it appears that exposing kids to more germs, microbes, and bacteria early in life might help them build up immunity.

Dr. Bock also finds the hygiene hypothesis persuasive, though he agrees with the December 9, 2008, *New York Times* article "Researchers Put a Microscope on Food Allergies," which states that "many researchers say the causes of food allergies are highly complex, and the 'hygiene hypothesis' cannot be the sole explanation." He points out that the proper balance of the immune system depends, among other things, on the right kinds of microbes and bacteria living in our intestines.

When I first started reading about the bacterial fauna living inside us, I was surprised to hear it called beneficial—I'd always thought of bacteria as a bad thing. But our digestion and our overall health actually depend on the right kind of bacteria and flora (microscopic plant life) flourishing in our gut.

So why don't our kids have enough friendly bacteria living inside them? Partly because they're not sufficiently exposed to nature. But partly because they're *over*exposed to antibiotics, which kill off both the dangerous bacteria and the friendly ones. And since scientists now believe that some 70 percent of our immune system is located in our intestines, our immune system isn't getting the beneficial bacteria that it needs in order to thrive.

"People need to be exposed to good intestinal bacteria," says Dr. Bock. "Basically, in our sterile society, there are tons of antibiotics wiping out all the microbes—including the good ones. People are not in the country playing in the dirt. . . . So we are not getting those kinds of exposures that we used to get in the old days."

I thought of how many rounds of antibiotics my four kids had been on before the age of five, and compared that to how rarely my brother, my sisters, and I had been given meds. I could see what the doctor meant. Then I asked him if the antibiotic overload was also due to the medications that can now be found in our food, especially in our meat, poultry, and dairy products.

Dr. Bock agreed that this was yet another assault on our friendly bacteria—and another possible cause of the allergy epidemic. (We'll learn more about antibiotics in milk in chapter 4.) My stomach sank as I realized that the very milk, meat, and medicine that I'd given my children to strengthen them might actually be causing them harm.

But at least Dr. Bock's explanations were making sense—far more sense than the more conventional version of the hygiene hypothesis, which seemed to suggest that our kids were getting sick because we kept our houses too clean. The very term "hygiene hypothesis" conjures up an image of hysterical housewives and manic mothers, a whole generation of women whose anxious devotion to Lysol and Purell was putting their kids at risk.

If you listen to the conventional wisdom of many doctors, pediatricians, and allergists, this version of the hygiene hypothesis is exactly what you'll hear. Although they don't come right out and say it, it's not too hard to read between the lines: they're saying that we moms are the problem. If we'd only lighten up on the hand-washing, they suggest, the allergy epidemic would vanish right into that new layer of dust covering our formerly spotless floors.

This theory played right into my Mama Guilt. But something didn't sit right. After the craziness of having four children in five years, my house often looked as though a bomb had just hit it. Excessive cleanliness was hardly a problem: not only was my house covered with a layer of dirt, but most times so were my kids! I could never figure out a way to get the kids to Purell their hands without immediately rubbing the alcohol into their eyes, so I'd given up on disinfectant when Lexy was a toddler. And while I'm not proud of the ketchup on my curtains or the blue yogurt stain on the ceiling (my husband and I still aren't sure how it got there), the fact remains: Tory had probably been exposed to every form of dust, dirt, and booger known to humankind before she was three months old.

Obviously, that's not science. But you don't have to rely on what a researcher would call my personal anecdotal evidence. The contradiction in the hygiene hypothesis is also acknowledged by some of our most prominent food allergy experts. For example, in "Food Allergies for Dummies," Dr. Wood writes that "some of the highest rates of asthma and allergies are in the inner city where hygiene is often no better than in undeveloped countries."

That seemed like an unwarranted dig at inner-city moms, but it made me stop and think. Although I'd never lived in the inner city, I did grow up in Houston, one of the nation's most polluted cities. If I'd been exposed to one level of environmental toxins, kids living near the area's factories, landfills, and oil refineries were obviously exposed to far worse. In fact, children growing up in poor urban neighborhoods are routinely exposed to exhaust, cigarettes, factory smoke, and a host of other toxic substances. Clearly, cleanliness per se is not the problem—antibiotics and pollutants are.

So here's my proposal, on behalf of moms and dads everywhere. If kids are getting allergies and asthma across the country, across the social classes, and across the racial divide, let's stop calling it the "hygiene hypothesis," as though somehow the problem was that we parents have gone overboard with the housekeeping (if only!). Instead, let's start calling it the "environmental hypothesis," to remind us that antibiotics in our food and toxins in the environment are probably part of the problem.

Oh, and one more thing: if antibiotics and environmental toxins are leading to the kind of immune-system imbalance that Dr. Bock talks about, and if they are indeed overstressing some vulnerable immune systems, producing unprecedented rates of asthma in inner-city kids as well as skyrocketing rates of allergies throughout the nation, *what the hell are they doing to the rest of us?*

Just asking.

The Allergy Epidemic and Our Food Supply

Sorry, folks, but I'm not quite done with the bad news yet. In my two-year quest to figure out what's behind the allergy epidemic, I went a bit beyond the box to look not just at the environment as a whole but also at changes in the food environment. So I turned to the work of two widely respected scientists, best-selling author Joel Fuhrman, MD, and Harvard researcher David Ludwig, MD.

Although these physicians have somewhat different approaches, both agree that changes in our food supply as well as our eating habits are creating serious threats to our health. Their theories are often ignored by an older generation of doctors, who were trained to focus on mainstream medical issues and tend to ignore the importance of nutrition. (If you really want to be left slack-jawed, ask your pediatrician or pediatric allergists how many hours they spent studying nutrition in medical school. Chances are you have read more about this subject than they have!) Younger and more innovative doctors, however, are beginning to grant nutrition the importance it deserves, and they may be more receptive to the ideas of these two pioneering researchers.

Dr. Fuhrman is the author of the best-selling *Eat for Health,* a two-volume guide to healthy eating that's being marketed to hospitals, doctors' offices, schools, universities, and corporations. He's also the father of four young kids. In Dr. Fuhrman's opinion, the major problem in the American diet is our reliance on processed foods. By switching from natural to processed foods—which, like so many sleep-deprived moms, I did—we deprive ourselves of nutrients that are vital to our health.

Dr. Fuhrman points out we get two types of nutrients from our food: *macronutrients,* which contain calories and come in the form of fats, proteins, and carbohydrates, and *micronutrients,* which contain no calories and come in the form of vitamins, minerals, and phytochemicals, or other types of plant-based chemicals. In our nation's switch from natural to processed foods, we're still getting the fat, calories, and carbs, but we're not getting the nutritional building blocks that we need. Even if processed foods are fortified with vitamins and minerals, they can't possibly be as good for us as natural foods, since we don't yet know all the micronutrients that these natural foods might hold.

As evidence, Dr. Fuhrman points to the steadily rising rates of disease since 1935, including cancer, autoimmune diseases, autism, and psychological diseases. He blames this increase on the fact that only 4 percent of the average American diet consists of what he calls "real food": vegetables, beans, nuts, seeds, fruits, and other natural items. Some 80 percent of our calories come from white flour, sugar, and oil, he points out, while some 60 percent of our calories come from processed foods that contain no micronutrients whatsoever—not even supplements of the vitamins and minerals we've already discovered, let alone any of the phytochemicals and micronutrients that we've yet to identify.

Dr. Fuhrman relates this overall health problem to the global rise of allergies. Although, as I mentioned earlier, there aren't good studies on the United States specifically, the International Study of Asthma and Allergies in Childhood has found that the global incidence of childhood allergies, asthma, and eczema increased by 0.5 percent annually from 1990 to 2003. By my calculations, 0.5 percent a year for thirteen years adds up to a nearly 7 percent total increase.

As we've seen, asthma is rising rapidly, in the United States as well as internationally, so that, according to 2005 data from the American Academy of Allergy, Asthma and Immunology, approximately 20 million Americans have asthma, or almost 10 percent of the population. And according to the Centers for Disease Control, some one in eight U.S. children suffers from asthma.

"Asthma *is* an allergy," remarks Dr. Fuhrman. "We shouldn't *be* so hypersensitive. Why are these diseases increasing so rapidly?" He cites poor diet, artificial substances in our diets, and overexposure to vaccines at an age when the immune system is still very vulnerable as the major culprits. His solution—and if we lived in a perfect world, maybe we could all swing it—is an organic, natural diet heavy in fruits, vegetables, nuts, and seeds.

Now, if your house is like mine, you may find Dr. Fuhrman's recom-

mendations challenging, to say the least. I know that given our budget constraints, allergy constraints, and flat-out temper tantrums by my toddlers,
my own family couldn't manage to go as far as Dr. Fuhrman feels is necessary. But for people struggling with obesity, autoimmune disorders, and
other inflammatory conditions, and for children whose allergies don't respond to less drastic measures, his dietary prescriptions might be a gift.

With Dr. Fuhrman's knowledge in hand, I turned to a Harvard doctor
who is also addressing our children's health. Dr. Ludwig is an associate
professor of pediatrics at Harvard Medical School and runs the Optimal
Weight for Life (OWL) clinic at Children's Hospital Boston—one of the
oldest and largest hospital-based programs for overweight children and
their families. He's the author of *Ending the Food Fight: Guide Your Child
to a Healthy Weight in a Fast Food, Fake Food World* and maintains the related Web site, www.endingthefoodfight.com.

Like Dr. Fuhrman, Dr. Ludwig is concerned about the U.S. dietary
shift away from natural foods and toward processed foods, which he goes
so far as to call "fake foods," and he too advocates "a diverse array of natural foods, rich in vitamins, minerals, antioxidants, and phytochemicals"—all those important nutritional building blocks that Dr. Fuhrman
talked about.

In fact, Dr. Ludwig believes that the shift to "fake food" has actually
altered our immune system. "And that," he told me, "more than any single chemical, may be behind the possible increase in food allergies, food
sensitivities, and food-related disorders." This made immediate sense to
me. Maybe we could call it the "fake-food hypothesis"!

Although many people respond adversely to specific additives and
preservatives found in processed foods (a topic we'll discuss further in
chapter 6), Dr. Ludwig is less concerned about any single ingredient than
about the overall effect of the scores of artificial ingredients that now
permeate our food supply. While a "small minority" of people might react
badly to a particular additive or preservative, he points out, "the greater
concern is how all of these substances interact over the long term," with
our bodies and with one another.

Dr. Ludwig's work raised all sorts of new questions in my mind. Okay, so one or two chemicals might not have much of an impact. But what happens when our food is loaded with so many chemicals that we now get a chemical cocktail in every bite?

Meanwhile, Dr. Ludwig explains, "the declining quality of children's diets is robbing them of the key vitamins, minerals, antioxidants, and plant chemicals that are known to support cellular metabolism and promote optimal health."

Perhaps, Dr. Ludwig suggests, this poor diet is affecting our immune system's ability to protect us. "Consuming a highly processed, very poor quality diet with too many of the wrong kinds of calories and not the right nutrients could dysregulate the immune system, just as poor nutrition has been well established to increase the risk for heart disease and diabetes. This dysregulation is either causing us to be less resistant to certain kinds of infections . . . or [to be] oversensitive . . . such as with food allergies or possibly even autoimmune disorders."

Either way, it seems, the "fake food" hitting our digestive tracts—where some scientists have speculated that much of our immune system is found—could be sabotaging our system. Sure, these fake foods are providing calories, chemicals, and convenience. But if they are making our kids sick, how convenient is that?

So there you have it. While many experts hesitate to discuss the potential causes behind the allergy epidemic, I've come to believe that there *are* some answers, which include four major factors:

1. The shift from a natural to an industrialized environment.
2. Excessive exposure to antibiotics, both as prescribed to our children and as consumed through antibiotic-laden meat, milk, and poultry.
3. The rise in pollutants and environmental toxins (perhaps including the fumes and residues from some of the chemical products we use to clean our homes).
4. Our tendency to eat more processed foods loaded with chemical additives and preservatives and to eat far fewer natural whole foods.

As I thought about these answers, I felt a sense of relief, but also a sense of responsibility. Suddenly, that after-school snackpack didn't seem quite as convenient as I thought. Maybe a banana was a better way to go.

Blurry Days and Milky Nights

As the winter of 2006 wore on, I felt as though I was moving faster than a sped-up cartoon character. I was working with my sister-in-law, a product development specialist, to create our new AllergyKids line, and drawing on the help of my Web designer brother-in-law to set up our Web site. Meanwhile, I was still a full-time mom caring for four little kids.

I'd kept on buying organic baby food for Tory, feeling that if her immune system was stressed, she should be getting the cleanest food possible. When she turned one, she was officially ready for milk, so I started buying her the organic stuff. As before, she got that while the rest of us got regular.

But one day in the dairy aisle, I had a thought. Why would I get special "clean" milk for Tory, and regular—presumably less clean—milk for my other kids. That didn't sit right.

I felt at first that I couldn't afford to buy organic milk for the whole family—it simply cost too much. But that didn't sit right, either. If something costs more, I reasoned, that's usually because it's better quality. So why is Tory getting the "good stuff" while the rest of my kids are making do with "second-rate"?

Let me tell you, switching to organic milk was one expense that I did *not* want to take on. Colin and John were like little milk-guzzling SUVs, drinking two and sometimes three glasses of milk each night before bed and countless more during the day. As I ferried an endless assortment of sippy cups back and forth between the fridge and the boys' bedroom, I came to feel like the milkwoman! But Jeff and I talked it over, and we agreed to spend the extra money.

If my nights were milky, my days were blurry with activity as the new business approached its Mother's Day launch date. I felt that I'd done everything I could to protect Tory in our house. Now I had to turn my efforts toward protecting her "out there." I wanted my kid to be able to go anywhere in the world and know that she was going to be safe. If we could get the word out on food allergies, make everyone aware of the problem, and maybe even fund a cure, then I would have done my job.

So I did my best to dot all the i's and cross all the t's for my new venture. Even though I was an MBA and had already helped found two companies, I had never entered the world of patents and trademarks, which everyone I spoke with insisted that I must do in order to protect the originality of my concept and symbol. So I turned to a bighearted local attorney who generously walked me through the whole process of trademarking, registration, and all the other things a new business requires. I also came up with our slogan: "Until there's a cure, there's AllergyKids."

This slogan was not only catchy, it was very close to my heart. After all, it was my little girl who was allergic. I didn't want her to rely on EpiPens (shots of either adrenaline or antihistamines administered in response to allergic reactions), and I didn't want her to spend a lifetime avoiding eggs. With a depth of passion that now seems almost naïve, I wanted nothing less than a cure.

Early on, I also decided that I needed the support of the medical and scientific communities as well. After all, a primary goal of AllergyKids would be to promote understanding of food allergies. I wasn't a doctor or a scientist, so I needed the guidance of people who were.

As it happened, one of the most prominent pediatric allergists in the nation, Dr. Allan S. Bock (no relation to Kenneth Bock), practiced right in my own city of Boulder—in fact, he's the one who finally diagnosed Tory's egg allergy. He was also on the board of the Food Allergy and Anaphylaxis Network (FAAN), the oldest and largest food allergy nonprofit in the country.

I was thrilled to have a nationally recognized expert as my child's doctor and decided that I should solicit his opinion as I launched Allergy-Kids. I wanted to show him that I respected his time, so I made a paying appointment with him, just as if I'd been a patient. I walked into his office with my armful of folders—my entire business plan and all my backup materials—and laid out my vision for him.

He was a buttoned-up man in a bow tie and glasses, and I remember that the whole time I was talking, he hardly looked me in the eyes. Finally, when I was finished, he looked up.

"There's no way I could be part of this," he said to me. "You know that I'm on the medical board of FAAN, so this would be a conflict of interest."

"But I'm trying to raise money for FAAN," I protested. "They're the group doing all the promotion—and I understand that they support food allergy research, too. Any funds I get, I plan to channel through them."

He just kept shaking his head. "Sorry," he kept saying. "It would be a conflict of interest."

I was stunned. How could there be a conflict of interest when it came to protecting the lives of children? Weren't we all trying to support research and the spread of information? Wasn't I a member of FAAN? I just didn't understand.

I called my husband as soon as I left the office. "How'd it go?" he asked.

Typically, I blamed myself. "I must not have explained it right," I said into my cell phone, trying not to sound as disappointed as I felt. "He said that my work represents a conflict of interest for him. I'll just have to get some more facts together. Maybe when the business has gotten off the ground, I'll go back and try again." I paused. "Jeff, do *you* see any conflict of interest?"

I could hear Jeff giving this problem the same thoughtful attention he brought to bear on everything, whether it had been buying our first home or whether we should try big-boy pants on Colin.

"No," he said finally, "I don't. But go back and try again, Robyn. Why not?"

Whenever I've been presented with an obstacle, my reaction is always to go back to the drawing board and work harder. So though I was thrown by the doctor's unexpected reaction, I was still absorbed in the start-up process for AllergyKids.

As it happened, a nationwide campaign called Food Allergy Awareness Week coincided with Mother's Day, and since I was a mother as well as a new business owner, I had decided to roll out the company right around that time. I sent out as many press releases as I could, primarily to local media but also to some national outlets. The food allergy epidemic was just beginning to reach the public's attention, and I guess local reporters liked the idea of a mother of four who was trying to help solve the problem, because I got a terrific response.

Unfortunately, the response from FAAN was not so terrific. I kept reaching out to them in a variety of ways, but I wasn't exactly getting a warm welcome. At the time, I was working with mothers around the country who, through FAAN, were sponsoring walks to raise money and awareness for the allergy issue. Hearing about my business, these mothers had come to me asking for financial donations for the Walk for the Cure fund-raisers that FAAN relied upon.

Starting up AllergyKids had taken every spare nickel we had. So I didn't have any cash, but I donated as many of our products as I could to show my support for these remarkable women around the country. I thought our company's products could perhaps be used as prizes for the top fund-raisers, or maybe they could be raffled off.

At the same time, I was sending periodic e-mails and letters to FAAN, asking if there was some way our two groups could work together. The women I worked with were happy with my contributions. But I never got a response from FAAN.

After a while, it occurred to me that money talks, and that FAAN might be more receptive if I sent them an actual donation. So I took a deep breath, dug deep, and mailed out a check.

Still no response. I knew that FAAN had formed partnerships with other allergy-related businesses, including one that sold EpiPens, so I didn't understand why they seemed to be giving me the cold shoulder. In what I now think of as the Mommy Mind-set—routinely deferring to authority—I blamed myself. As I had when I met the pediatric allergist, I thought, *I must just not be explaining myself properly.*

Mother's Day and the Mommy Mind-set: I (Reluctantly) Start to Question Authority, Part 1

My Mommy Mind-set was in full swing when I got a confusing e-mail from one of FAAN's public relations people in Washington, D.C. The official congratulated me for a local TV news appearance—I guess she was one of the seven or eight people who actually watched the early morning local broadcast that Saturday—but took me to task for saying that there was "no universal program out there" designed to address the food allergy issue.

But I hadn't said that. What I'd said was that there was no universal *symbol* for food allergies, which there wasn't. Other than AllergyKids' green stop sign with the exclamation point in the center, there still isn't. So I was surprised that she'd go to all that trouble to watch my broadcast and then mistake what I had said.

But second, and more important, I was a bit taken aback at receiving this four-paragraph official-sounding e-mail from the organization that I had been trying so hard—and so fruitlessly—to connect with. Reading between the lines, what I heard was, "We're the major food allergy non-profit—you're just a small local company. When it comes to press and promotion, let us take the lead." Were they trying to tell me to stick to my bake sales?

Still in the Mommy Mind-set, I thought that I just had to explain myself better. So I responded with an e-mail that was as inviting—and as open-ended—as I could make it:

> We would be thrilled to work with your organization, as we are engaging partners across the non-profit, business and medical communities. How would you propose that we work together?

I never heard a thing.

I did hear, however, from CNN, which invited me to appear on the air on Father's Day weekend. They wanted to do something to acknowledge the growing allergy epidemic, and they liked the idea of a mother of four starting a business for parents and their allergic kids. Despite a few minor traumas—the power went out on our block the morning of my appearance, and I had to do my first live national TV show without so much as a shower—the program went well.

Allergies were becoming a hot topic, so a few weeks later I was asked to appear on ABC national news as well. I was thrilled with the boost it would give my struggling new business and delighted to think I was helping to promote awareness of food allergies for the millions of kids like Tory who had to struggle with their condition every day. Although I didn't expect clear sailing, I was feeling optimistic.

Then a series of bewildering events occurred that to this day I don't fully understand. First, one of the women sponsoring a fund-raising walk for FAAN asked the group on my behalf, without my knowledge, if it would lend its name to AllergyKids as a sponsor. I don't know why she did that, and, perhaps not surprisingly, FAAN wrote back to her, saying that they'd deal with me directly. The woman forwarded me the correspondence, and I wasn't quite sure what to do.

Then, in August, I took part in a conference call with that woman and another who was also sponsoring a FAAN walk. One of them told me that in a recent call with FAAN, AllergyKids had actually been on the agenda. That struck me as strange, as the group had yet to respond to a single one of my letters or e-mails on ways that we could work together. So I asked the two women to elaborate.

"They're saying that you took copyrighted material from the organization," one of them said. "I think they're going to sue you."

My heart stopped. *What?*

The woman helpfully sent me a copy of the e-mail that FAAN had distributed to many of its top volunteers, including, of course, women I was working with and with whom I hoped to establish long-term relationships in this important work for our children. Since that e-mail is the property of FAAN, I can't quote it here, but it basically accused me of copying some of FAAN's materials without permission and said that the group was planning to send me a cease-and-desist letter. Volunteers were also told that FAAN didn't endorse, promote, or recommend AllergyKids or its Web site, and that it wouldn't accept our sponsorship or our donations.

After sending FAAN money, donating thousands of dollars in products, and repeatedly attempting to engage them in my efforts, what could I possibly have done to have merited this response? I was baffled—and, I'll admit it, more than a little hurt. But most of all, I was struggling with the Mommy Mind-set, because I kept wondering what I had done to provoke this powerful group.

Eventually, I received the cease-and-desist letter, which I immediately brought to my lawyer. The so-called copying concerned our slogan, which appears on our Web site, our products, and all our e-mails: "Until there's a cure, there's AllergyKids." According to FAAN, this wording was far too close to a phrase that they themselves had used in an annual report from 2004: "Until there is a cure, education is the key."

Wait a minute—they were upset about our *slogan*? But that sentence had been approved and trademarked by the U.S. Patent and Trademark Office. If it had truly belonged to someone else, the government would have let me know.

My bighearted lawyer was also a bulldog, so as soon as he saw FAAN's mass e-mail, he wanted to sue FAAN for defamation and loss of income. After all, I was counting on my reputation to develop the relationships I needed to promote my company and earn funds for the cause. I couldn't do either if people thought I was a thief.

More important, the slogan clearly had not been stolen. "Until there's a cure" was hardly the property of FAAN. The Until There's a Cure Foundation had taken the phrase for its very name. The Peanut Allergy Foundation of Maine also used the slogan, "Until there's a cure." An assisted living facility in Delaware used the tag line, "Until there's a cure, there's Somerford Place." In fact, my lawyer's Google search on August 7, 2006, turned up more than 27,000 hits for the phrase.

But to my lawyer's dismay, I didn't want to get into a legal battle. First, I couldn't afford to—AllergyKids was already taking every spare penny and every spare minute. Second, I wanted to figure out why this was happening. What had I done to threaten FAAN so? Why were they having an allergic reaction to *me*?

In order to find out what was causing the food allergy epidemic, I'd become a kind of detective. Now, to find out what was motivating FAAN, I would have to turn my detecting skills from science to politics. It wasn't a task that I ever would have chosen. But somehow, this task had chosen me.

Collecting Corporate Cash

As with so many aspects of this journey, I actually stumbled into my first discovery by accident. I was speaking with one of the "allergy moms" who had heard about my cease-and-desist letter. She said, "Well, a lot of people don't agree with the way FAAN does business. You know, they take money from Kraft."

That's weird, I thought. Like every busy American mom, I knew Kraft primarily as the wonderful company that made instant and affordable mac 'n' cheese for my kids. I appreciated the product, which I bought in bulk at Costco and which my kids could always be counted on to scarf down, but I couldn't see why Kraft would want to fund food allergy research or education.

Hoping to learn more, I went hunting for a mention of Kraft on the FAAN Web site—maybe among its funders, or was there a list of corporate sponsors? Nope. Nothing. *Odd.*

Then I looked on the Kraft Web site. Bingo. On the Kraft Corporate Social Responsibility page was a little note that in 1998, Kraft had started funding the FAAN Web site and had been its sole sponsor ever since.

Wait a minute. Its *sole* sponsor? That was a heck of a lot of influence for one major food corporation to have. In business school, I'd had this wonderful ethics professor who taught us always to ask, "What incentive does a corporation have for doing something?" What incentive did Kraft have for funding FAAN? And what incentive did FAAN have to not disclose this funding? Would I have felt the same way about the information they provided if the Kraft logo and full disclosure had appeared on FAAN's Web site?

Now, let me be very clear. I'm not saying that FAAN should not have taken the money. I'm saying that they should have made it public that they were doing so. Two years later, when I was raising questions about the role of processed foods and soy additives in the food allergy epidemic, FAAN's experts pooh-poohed my claim. Of course, that's their right. But wouldn't their arguments have looked different if it had been public knowledge that they were being funded by a manufacturer of processed food that uses soy additives?

If Kraft was so proud of funding the FAAN Web site, why was there no mention by FAAN of the Kraft connection? By the way, since I started raising these issues, Kraft removed the mention of its funding from its Web site, though, as of fall 2006, it was still there. And when I was profiled in a 2008 *New York Times* article in which I publicly highlighted the Kraft connection, FAAN suddenly decided that their Web site should be funded by an entirely different organization. It's now supported by a grant from the American College of Allergy, Asthma and Immunology (ACAAI), a nonprofit group of medical personnel working in the allergy-immunology field.

However, the ACAAI's own Web site has a corporate connection. It used to be sponsored by Dura Pharmaceuticals, a company that develops and markets prescription pharmaceutical products for the treatment of allergies, asthma, and other respiratory ailments. Now it's sponsored by AstraZeneca, one of the world's leading pharmaceutical companies. So clearly, Big Food and Big Pharma have an interest in overseeing the research and promotion of allergy-related information.

In fact, the more I looked into FAAN's business, the more corporate connections I kept uncovering. In addition to the Kraft connection, here's a summary of what I found:

• The Peanut Foundation, a group sponsored by the peanut industry, funded at least three research projects whose principal investigator was FAAN executive director, Anne Munoz-Furlong.

The first project ran from 1999 to 2000, a $14,000 endeavor
called "Educate the Educator." It was intended to teach principals, nurses, and dieticians in U.S. schools about how to manage
students who suffered from peanut allergies—obviously, a worthwhile goal—but it also reflected the industry's point of view. "The
decision makers and parents should also be educated that bans
do not work," says the project summary. Not exactly a neutral position when you consider how much revenue would be at stake if
a peanut butter ban were suddenly to be implemented in school
lunchrooms across the country. I could understand why the industry was taking that position—but why was the head of a major
food allergy group? And how would the group's members, many of
whom *did* support a ban, feel if they knew?

The second project, also intended to "help educate education
personnel," ran from 2000 to 2001, with a $15,875 grant, and also
with Ms. Furlong as principal investigator. The third project for
$13,000, ran from 2005 to 2006, also with Ms. Munoz-Furlong,
also to "increase awareness of food allergy and anaphylaxis among
school staff." It seemed pretty clear to me that the Peanut Foundation wanted some say over how school personnel dealt with the
allergy issue—but why was the head of the major food allergy nonprofit taking money to help promote the industry's point of view?
Even if she legitimately agreed with their approach, shouldn't the
relationship have been publicized on FAAN's Web site so FAAN
members could decide for themselves what they thought of this
connection?

• The Center for Science in the Public Interest (CSPI) is a
watchdog organization that seeks to maintain integrity in research
by highlighting relationships between research and funding. It reports that in 2001 FAAN sponsored a Web site for teenagers and
children "funded by an educational grant from Dey, L.P.," called

FAANKids. Dey makes the EpiPen—the device that parents of allergic and asthmatic kids use to protect their children from anaphylactic shock. The company was also an associate of Merck KGaA, a German corporation that makes medications for allergies and respiratory diseases.

So now, along with Big Food, we had Big Pharma putting its stamp on FAAN's Web sites. I'm not saying that the pharmaceutical companies shouldn't promote their own point of view. But why was the major food allergy nonprofit helping them do so?

• FAAN medical board member A. Wesley Burks, Jr., is listed as one of the inventors of a patented peanut allergen—part of research being done to develop a nonallergenic peanut. Another inventor listed on the same patent is Gary A. Bannon, who was affiliated with the University of Arkansas where Burks had also conducted research and later an employee of the Monsanto Corporation, one of the largest chemical corporations in the world. Monsanto (whom we'll look at more closely in coming chapters) also produces genetically modified seeds, as well as pesticides, insecticides, and other agricultural products.

When I started to think about it, this connection made my head spin. FAAN board members were working with a major corporation to develop a potentially profitable food product. Again, not that they shouldn't have done so. But shouldn't they have let us know about this corporate connection?

• In another Monsanto tie, FAAN medical board member Hugh Sampson was listed as coauthor with Gary Bannon and other company researchers on numerous research articles on peanut allergies. According to the U.S. Patent and Trademark Office, Sampson was even listed as a coinventor on a new Monsanto protein designed to make plants more insect-resistant.

• According to notes dated July 2005 from the Peanut Genome Initiative, a group of international scientists committed to "meet the needs of the peanut industry through genomics and biotechnology" (whose members include Kraft and the United States Department of Agriculture), it also appeared that Sampson and Burks were analyzing the cross-reactivity between the soybean and the peanut—the ways that people who were allergic to one might also be allergic to the other. In fact, Sampson and Burks (a steering committee member of the Peanut Genome Initiative) had been granted $17 million to conduct research for the Peanut Genome Initiative.

• According to the *Journal of Nutrition,* my bespectacled and bow-tied pediatric allergist, Dr. Allan S. Bock—the one who'd refused to work with me for fear of conflict of interest—had conducted research in 1988 in which he testified to the safety of MSG (monosodium glutamate), a controversial soy-derived additive used in processed foods to enhance flavor. The research had been conducted with Hugh Sampson, Robert Zeiger, and other members of FAAN's board.

• The chairman of the board of FAAN was a man named Joseph Levitt, the former director of the FDA's Center for Food Safety and Applied Nutrition. I also learned that thirty years ago he had drafted an influential memo for the FDA that led to the acceptance of a controversial artificial sweetener called aspartame, which was manufactured by a Monsanto subsidiary—and that the FDA had been refusing to approve. (Aspartame is used in making NutraSweet and Equal.)

When I first discovered these connections, I didn't quite know what to make of them. But I was beginning to realize that the nonprofit world, our government's regulatory agencies, and the corporations who produced food, seeds, pesticides, and insecticides were all involved with one another in intimate, if not downright unhealthy, ways. I was reminded of the words of French political thinker Alexis de Tocqueville, often quoted by Monsanto, that "the public will always believe a simple lie rather than a complex truth."

I had always thought of FAAN as an objective organization whose only goal was to help kids with allergies. But its board and staff now seemed to be full of people with corporate connections. Although I had believed that our government was completely dedicated to protecting all Americans, I now began to wonder whether corporate interests mattered more than children's health. I had believed we were all on the same side— working to protect children and solve the food allergy crisis. But now I was beginning to have my doubts. And as much as I did not want to wonder about these issues, somehow they wouldn't go away.

3

SOY SECRETS

By August 2006, I felt that things had finally settled into a kind of equilibrium. AllergyKids had been in business for three months, and while I felt as though I hadn't slept since the January evening when I first conceived of the company, we seemed to have successfully completed the launch of what I was now calling my fifth baby.

I'd also figured out how to police the egg exposure at the kitchen table, somehow managing to keep the family fed without exposing Tory to eggs. I'd come up with a lot of little tricks to keep her away from processed foods—not because I was worried about additives or preservatives or even nutrition, but because I could never be sure whether a processed food contained eggs since eggs often went by the code names of "albumin," "globulin," or "livetin" on the label. Was that even English?

So, for example, when I cooked up some of Kraft's bright-orange mac 'n' cheese for my family, I gave Tory the noodles only, none of that sauce made from the little packet of powder. I had nothing against the sauce, which I happily fed to Lexy, Colin, and John two or three nights a week—I just didn't know what was in it. So none for Tory; more for the rest of us!

I've since learned that frustrations with labeling are a common theme among allergy parents. It's very difficult to get companies to label packages clearly, identifying the most common allergens under names you can recognize. Milk protein, for example, is called "casein," so that's a "danger word" that milk-allergy parents need to recognize. Likewise, any word beginning with "malto" signals a corn product, and so on. To identify all the danger elements in ordinary foods, allergy parents practically need an advanced course in chemistry.

Luckily, labeling laws are getting better, thanks to the Center for Science in the Public Interest. Under the direction of executive director Michael Jacobson, PhD, the group spearheaded the passage of the Food Allergen Labeling and Consumer Protection Act, which went into effect January 2006, and which requires that foods containing the top eight allergens must declare these ingredients in plain language on the ingredients list or meet other types of labeling requirements.

Unfortunately, loopholes in the list still make it hard for allergy parents to protect their kids. Companies have a powerful incentive to be as vague as possible about the inclusion of potential allergens in their products so that if kids have an allergic reaction, parents will find it harder to sue. I'm not saying that corporations are acting maliciously. But I do believe that most of them would prefer to avoid situations where they might be held legally accountable for something that could be the basis of a lawsuit.

This issue of labeling, which seemed almost trivial to me prior to Tory's first allergic reaction, now seems to me of paramount importance—and not only for allergy parents, either. According to a November 21, 2008, investigative report by the *Chicago Tribune,* "In effect, children are used as guinea pigs, with the government and industry often taking steps to properly label a product only after a child has been harmed." The investigation also "revealed that the government rarely inspects food to find problems and doesn't punish companies that repeatedly violate labeling laws."

Here are some figures from that article, entitled "Children at Risk in Food Roulette: Mislabeling, Lax Oversight Threaten People with Allergies":

- 47 percent of products recalled for hidden allergens since 1998 were not announced to the public
- an average of five products each week are recalled because of hidden allergens
- one-third of these products are cookies, candy, ice cream, or snacks
- 50 percent of allergen recalls involve undisclosed milk or eggs in a product

According to the article, "in many cases, the government and companies never inform consumers." The *Tribune* found that nearly half of the allergy-related recalls in the last ten years were not announced to the public. This was true even in dozens of cases where the FDA classified products as likely to cause serious harm or death.

As a parent of children with allergies, I find this article chilling. All of us have the right to know what's in our kids' food and to make informed decisions about whether we want to ply them with hormone-laden milk or genetically engineered soy. We need to know that soy is in a thousand places we might never expect it, often in the form of "vegetable oil" (found in salad dressings, soup, and imitation meat products, for starters), and that high-fructose corn syrup lurks in foods that don't seem "corny" to us: breads, ketchup, granola bars, and even English muffins.

As I've come to know more about food, I've also learned about the potential hazards of genetic engineering—information that I'll share with you in this chapter and the next two—which has made me feel even more strongly about labeling laws. We deserve to know which foods contain this new altered DNA so that we can decide for ourselves whether we want our kids to take part in this massive science experiment. How can we choose wisely when the food we buy isn't even labeled?

All of Europe and Great Britain, Australia, Japan, and even Russia have very strong labeling laws, requiring food manufacturers to make perfectly clear when a product contains genetically engineered ingredients. And several African countries, including Algeria, Benin, Ghana, and Zambia, have a "no-genetic-engineering" policy for their domestic market, while even more—Angola, Malawi, Mozambique, Namibia, Nigeria, Sudan, and Zimbabwe—have refused even to accept unmilled genetically modified grain as food aid. Are we U.S. consumers really so much more ignorant or so much less concerned about our kids' food? As an American, I'm offended by that idea, and I hope you are, too.

But back in the summer of 2006, I hadn't gotten there yet. I was still just going along as I always had, tweaking Tory's diet to remove the processed food, serving up the blue yogurt and dinosaur-shaped chicken nuggets to everybody else.

Then I happened to catch an episode of *Good Morning, America* in which Diane Sawyer was hosting a report called "Secrets in Your Food," about children's foods that contain genetically modified ingredients. I had never heard of GMOs (genetically modified organisms), GE (genetically engineered) foods, or any of the other acronyms. In fact, at first I thought GMOs were a kind of nutritional supplement, maybe like Omegas. But as the television squawked that morning, the idea of DNA fragments in my kids' snackpacks started to give me chills.

As I watched the program, I became more and more disturbed. I had no idea that so many ingredients in my kids' foods had been altered in this way. Even Diane Sawyer seemed surprised. At one point she looked out toward the crew and said something like, "Did you guys know you were eating this stuff?"

Apparently I wasn't the only one who hadn't heard about this issue. I was still doing lots of Google-based research on food allergies and had grown quite dependent on Google Alerts, which keep you up-to-date with the latest articles about any terms you request. "What's one more term?" I figured, so I typed in "GMO" and all the other initials that were associated with the process. Then I returned to the nonstop action of raising a family and running a business.

A few days later, something surprising popped up on my computer: a news report about a Michigan study exploring "the potential of genetically engineered foods to cause allergic reactions in humans."

What? How interesting! That was a connection I wasn't even looking for. But somehow, my quest to discover what lay behind the allergy epidemic and my new casual interest in GMOs had come together, purely as a matter of coincidence.

Or *was* it just coincidence? According to the press release from Michigan State University, GMOs were crops such as corn and soy whose DNA had been modified by the insertion of a protein from a different organism. The genetically engineered crops that resulted were supposed to be more resistant to insects or diseases.

By this time, I knew that food allergies were an overreaction to a protein that the immune system reads as foreign and dangerous. So learning about this study made me wonder whether the genetically engineered proteins added to corn and soy were being read as foreign by our kids' immune systems. Was *this* the trigger behind the new surge of allergic responses? Or perhaps these new proteins were another factor in the toxic food environment that Drs. Bock, Ludwig, and Fuhrman had described, one more strain on young immune systems that were already overly stressed by pollutants, toxins, and too many processed foods.

I began to wonder about a possible link between genetic engineering and food allergies. Imagine my surprise when I discovered that genetically altered soy had its first widespread use in 1996. Not only had some researchers discovered that soy contained approximately fifteen soybean proteins that could be recognized by soybean-sensitive people (the published reports of that research didn't clarify whether the scientists were investigating conventional soy or genetically engineered soy), but other researchers had found that levels of a major soy allergen, trypsin inhibitor, were 27 percent higher in genetically modified soy.

I knew that soy and peanuts were both legumes. Could these increased levels of soy allergens in this genetically engineered soy somehow be triggering the dramatic increase in peanut allergies? Was it just coincidence that peanut allergies had begun to rise by 20 percent each year starting in 1997, just after genetically modified soy was widely introduced? Were there any studies that might address this?

What about the fact that soy itself became one of the top eight U.S.

allergens just about the time that genetically modified (GM) soy was introduced to the United States? Was that a coincidence, too?

My antennae really went up when I learned that in 1998, the year that genetically modified soy was introduced in the United Kingdom, the U.K. rate of soy allergies jumped 50 percent. Was this just one coincidence too many?

That night, I stayed on the computer for hours. At midnight, Jeff came groggily down the stairs to say good night, but he woke up as soon as he saw my face. I guess he could see the energy burning through me that night, as I was torn between excitement over my discovery and horror over what I was learning.

"What's going on?" he asked.

"I think I've found something," I said, and told him about the connections I was making between the new proteins introduced by genetic engineering and the skyrocketing allergy epidemic. I reminded him that food allergies are basically an overreaction to a protein that the body perceives as a toxic invader and suggested that maybe our kids' immune systems were perceiving these new, lab-created proteins as precisely that.

"Do you think it's possible?" I asked. "Don't you think there might be a connection? I mean, look at all these studies—people have been talking about the link between genetic engineering and allergic reactions since at least 1994."

Jeff shook his head. "What do the experts say?"

"I don't know," I told him. "There's nothing about genetically modified organisms on the FAAN Web site or in any of the discussions of allergies that I've read. It looks as though the pediatric allergists haven't put two and two together—do you think that's possible?"

We stared at each other. It now seems incredible that we were so naïve, but we really did believe that perhaps others in the allergy community simply weren't aware of this link. I couldn't wait to share my discovery with the parents I'd been working with. And Jeff was so proud of me that the next day he brought me flowers.

Of course, I now know that lots of people in the allergy community were aware of these concerns. In fact, the nationally respected allergy specialists Dr. Hugh Sampson and Dr. A. Wesley Burks—both members of FAAN's medical board—had also written explicitly about the possible links between soy allergies and peanut allergies and had acknowledged the widespread presence in the U.S. food supply of genetically altered soy, corn, and other products. Dr. Sampson had even been part of an investigation into something called StarLink corn, a genetically engineered strain of cattle feed that had accidentally entered the human food supply, triggering life-threatening allergic reactions. (You can read more about the StarLink scandal in chapter 5.)

But there was not one word about genetic engineering on FAAN's Web site. Outside of the scientists whose articles I was now researching, no one in the allergy world seemed to be talking about the relationship between the widespread introduction of these genetically engineered proteins and the skyrocketing allergy epidemic.

Later I would learn that as these crops were initially introduced, respected pediatric allergists like Fred McDaniel Atkins, MD, who had also previously served on FAAN's medical board, had urged caution, based on his research into the allergenicity of genetically modified foods. I would even learn that Dr. Hugh Sampson, currently on FAAN's medical board, had taken part in a 2001 National Toxicology Program sponsored by the Department of Health and Human Services workshop entitled "Assessment of the Allergenic Potential of Genetically Modified Foods."

The issue had attracted international attention as well. For example, the Food and Agricultural Organization of the United Nations (FAO) and the U.N.'s World Health Organization (WHO) had sponsored a joint report on the allergenicity of genetically modified foods. Experts who helped prepare this report included former FAAN medical board member Steve Taylor, MD, and a slew of other doctors who were trying to figure out some way to assess the safety of these new proteins.

As you can see, I was hardly the first to be concerned about either genetic engineering or the possible connection between GMOs and the allergy epidemic. So why wasn't this front and center on the Web sites of FAAN and the other allergy sites I visited regularly? Why had all the pediatric allergists who served on the board of FAAN failed to inform parents of this issue on FAAN's Web site, even as they discussed it with their colleagues, with governmental officials, and with executives and researchers from the corporations who were manufacturing genetically altered crops?

Clearly, I wasn't the first to wonder about the connection between allergies and the genetic modification of our food supply. Nor was I the first to wonder about the humble little soybean, which, as I've learned, may pose a variety of health problems—even before the genetic engineers get their hands on it. When I found out about the hidden side of soy, I was astonished, upset—and relieved to finally have the truth. So in this chapter, I'll share all my soy secrets with you.

The Hidden Side of Soy

Like most moms who came of age during the 1980s and 1990s, I'd always heard that soy was good for you. I'd picked up the idea that this high-protein legume was a terrific alternative to red meats and even poultry— far less likely to boost cholesterol levels and much better for your heart.

I'd also heard that Asian women, with their high-soy diets, didn't even have a word for menopause, and that soy in all its forms was good for women's hormonal health and good for people's health in general. Wanting to do right by my children-to-be, I ate edamame (steamed soybeans) throughout my pregnancies. I was so proud when my oldest daughter, at the age of two, seemed to enjoy edamame as much as I did.

Little did I know that in 1998, two officials at the Food and Drug Administration (FDA) had expressed their concern about soy's possible health risks. Daniel M. Sheehan, PhD, was the director of the FDA's Estrogen Base Program in its Division of Genetic and Reproductive Toxicology. Daniel R. Doerge, PhD, was with the FDA's Division of Biochemical Toxicology. Both were disturbed by what they called the "abundant evidence" that soy had been found to cause a variety of prob-

lems in "estrogen-sensitive tissues," such as women's breasts and reproductive organs, and that it might also be toxic to the thyroid.

The heart of the problem, in the scientists' view, was soy's high con-
centration of *isoflavones,* a type of micronutrient that has a wide variety
of both positive and negative effects. Think of them as another version
of the good cop/bad cop routine.

On the "good cop" side, isoflavones are one of the most powerful antioxidants, which means they can help prevent aging, boost immunity,
and generally contribute to a sense of health and well-being. Isoflavones
also have a significant impact on estrogen, the female hormone, which
means that they might ease or prevent the symptoms of menopause and
contribute to women's hormonal health in a number of ways.

But that plus can also be a minus, turning our good cops bad, because
isoflavones' very ability to boost estrogen production can also pose hazards to our health. For example, the FDA scientists point out, during
pregnancy, isoflavones *could* boost estrogen levels even higher, which
"could be a risk factor for abnormal brain and reproductive tract development."

In women, excess production of estrogen has also been associated
with breast cancer and with other reproductive cancers. In boys, extra estrogen in utero can lead to testicular cancer and sometimes to such "male
problems" as undescended testicles and infertility.

When I read that, my heart was flooded with a double dose of Mama
Guilt, laced with a little pang of fear. So all that soy I'd eaten while I was
pregnant *hadn't* been good for my kids? And maybe it had put Colin and
John at risk for testicular cancer or infertility, while possibly exposing
Lexy, Tory, and me to a higher risk of breast or ovarian cancer?

But the bad news didn't end there. The FDA scientists went on to
warn that soy isoflavones might also cause "goitrogenic and even carcinogenic effects," meaning that they could produce goiter (a disease of
the thyroid gland) and even cancer. Both children and adults were at risk
for this effect, especially if the children had been fed soy formula when
they were infants.

This stopped me in my tracks, as so many "allergy babies" who'd been unable to tolerate cow's milk formula had been switched to soy formula as a substitute. It was devastating to think that in trying to protect kids from something they were allergic to, parents had inadvertently exposed their children to an even greater danger.

Wait a minute, I thought, wishing I didn't have to learn all this. *There has to be more. What about all those positive effects I'd read about—soy's supposed benefits to my heart and reproductive system?*

The doctors had an answer for that, too: "all estrogens which have been studied carefully in human populations are two-edged swords in humans . . . with both beneficial and adverse effects resulting from the administration of the same estrogen." Therefore, they concluded, although isoflavones themselves hadn't been studied in detail, "it is likely that [they share] the same characteristics."

Okay. So the jury was still out on soy. But since I wouldn't hand my kids a double-edged sword to play with, why had I inadvertently put one on the dinner table?

Even though the effect of isoflavones hasn't been extensively studied in humans, many animal experiments have been done. And, the scientists wrote, "The animal data is also consistent with adverse effects in humans." Not exactly a resounding vote of confidence!

I know it sounds confusing. Sometimes the problem is too much estrogen, and other times the problem is too little. But that's part of the mystery of isoflavones—they can act both to boost estrogen levels and to suppress them, and depending on the circumstances, either the boosting or the suppression might be positive—or negative. That's why the scientists called isoflavones a double-edged sword. The important point was that these FDA scientists thought soy wasn't safe, especially for infants, and they felt strongly enough about it to write to the FDA.

As it happens, the FDA didn't go along with the views of Sheehan and Doerge. In May–June 2000, an article in *FDA Consumer* magazine acknowledged the controversy but asserted that all the scientific evidence wasn't really in yet and promoted the health claims of soy, with particular emphasis on its benefits to heart health. The pro-soy article even included a list of suggestions for adding soy to your diet in the form of soy-based beverages, soy milk, and soy cheese.

But Doerge and Sheehan felt strongly enough about the issue to keep swimming upstream. In June 2002, they published an article in a journal called *Environmental Health Perspectives,* repeating their concern that soy isoflavones generated the production of estrogen and were potentially toxic to the thyroid. They called for further study, writing that "[r]igorous, high-quality experimental and human research is the best way to address these concerns."

Since that article was published, soy continues to be studied, though not to the extent that Sheehan and Doerge recommended. However, at least one prestigious medical organization has backed away from its former pro-soy position, though very few Americans are aware of its reversal. In 2006, the American Heart Association (AHA) conducted a review of twenty-two studies on the effects of soy protein with isoflavones, concluding that soy had "minimal or no benefit on cholesterol." As a result, an AHA committee "could not recommend the use of isoflavone supplements in pills or food for the prevention of heart disease." And indeed, the American Heart Association quietly withdrew its pro-soy claims.

Wait a minute. I remembered hearing about the American Heart Association's *support* for soy. Why hadn't I heard about its change of position? In all the busyness of motherhood, had I just missed the headlines?

My curiosity piqued, I went hunting for news coverage. Interestingly, I found some articles criticizing soy that had appeared several years ago, such as the January 26, 2000, *New York Times* article by health columnist Marian Burros: "Against the backdrop of widespread praise . . . there is growing suspicion that soy—despite its undisputed benefits—may pose some health hazards. . . . Not one of the 18 scientists interviewed for this column was willing to say taking isoflavones was risk free." But no more news about soy risk from the *New York Times* since then—and nothing about the AHA's 2006 reversal.

What about the *Washington Post*? In January 2001, the *Post* also urged caution in its Health Section: "You have to be soy careful: tofu and similar foods may be beneficial, but some experts fear that too much could be unsafe."

But then, again, nothing.

Wow. Had *anyone* in the mainstream media covered the AHA's withdrawal of its support for soy?

The only big story I found was the January 22, 2006, report on CBS News, "Soy May Not Lower Cholesterol: American Heart Association Says Soy May Not Ward Off Heart Disease," though CNN did mention the change in an article on its Web site as part of their weekly roundup of medical journals.

So if you, too, spent the last ten years believing that soy had all sorts of heart-healthy benefits and might have appreciated knowing that the American Heart Association no longer thinks it does—let alone if you would have liked to know something about the dangers of soy—I guess you had to be watching CBS on January 22, 2006. Or else you had to catch the one *Times* and the one *Post* story that ran several years ago. Perhaps there was simply too much other news to cover. Whatever the explanation, consumers remained uninformed that a major claim for soy's health benefits had now been withdrawn by one of the country's most respected health organizations.

And if you were pregnant, nursing, or feeding small children since those stories appeared? I guess, like me, you were just out of luck. And so, I guess, were your kids.

The Fat Fallacy: How Soy Affects Our Digestion

Another soy secret that I learned is the legume's tendency to block our absorption of essential minerals, including calcium, magnesium, phosphorus, copper, iron, and zinc. That's because soy is rich in phytic acid, a substance that interferes with mineral absorption.

Soy also contains toxins that interfere with the enzymes that we need for our digestion. One of our most important enzymes is called trypsin, essential to the digestion of protein, which, coincidentally, kids with food allergies have a problem with. According to respected nutritionists Sally Fallon and Mary G. Enig, PhD: "These toxins that act as inhibitors [within soy] are large, tightly folded proteins that are not completely de-activated during ordinary cooking. They can produce serious gastric distress, reduced protein digestion and chronic deficiencies in amino acid uptake. In test animals, diets high in trypsin inhibitors cause enlargement and pathological conditions of the pancreas, including cancer."

But what about the billions of people in Asia who have lived on soy for thousands of years? As it happens, other factors having to do with the Asian diet seem to negate some of these effects. Their cooking techniques—fermentation and precipitation—seem to counteract many of the worst effects of soy. Asians also tend to consume soy products along with meat or fish, so that, according to Fallon and Enig, "the mineral-blocking effects of the phytates are reduced."

Now, I grew up on red meat and potatoes in the south, so I've never eaten tofu. But I knew people who lived on it. And, as you just heard, one of the proudest days of my young motherhood was learning that my two-year-old Lexy shared my pleasure in steamed soybeans—I thought I was teaching her the joys of a healthy diet. So I found it thoroughly unsettling to read about the potentially harmful effects of traditional Asian foods.

But at least those methods of preparation counteracted some of the worst aspects of soy. I was even more disturbed to learn that soy's effects are far worse when it's consumed in the form of soy protein isolates, such as in soy milk, soy cheese, and soy hot dogs, or in the soy protein added to virtually every processed food on the market as well as to most protein bars and protein powders. As I thought about the allergy kids who relied on soy for their daily protein, I started to get a stomachache just reading these soy secrets.

Then I learned something that was even more fascinating—in a nauseating kind of way. Apparently, pigs also have trouble digesting soy. I read about this in a May 2003 American Soybean Association bulletin entitled "Correcting the Myths." The association was boasting about soy's benefits as livestock feed for multistomach animals, such as cows, but acknowledged that soy was "non-digestible" in animals who have only one stomach, such as pigs. Of course, we humans have only one stomach, too.

I wasn't sure I wanted to read about the digestive process of a pig. But if we were having the same problems digesting soybeans as they were, I guess I had to know. And the soybean industry spared me none of the gory details: "Instead of being digested in the stomach, [the soy] passes to the intestines where bacteria ferment it into gases that make animals feel full, and they can be discouraged from eating and gaining weight to their full genetic potential."

Well, there's a charming image. I pictured pigs scarfing down their daily ration of soybeans—and then stopping as their intestines became bloated and gassy. Yes, I could see how that might keep them from fattening up.

According to the bulletin, conventional soybeans contained too much of a carbohydrate called stachyose, which interferes with the piggies' digestion. So to help with the fattening process, the soybean industry had engineered a new type of soybean in which the hard-to-digest stachyose had been replaced by a gentler carb: "the easily digested sugar sucrose."

Hmmm. What do you think happens to pigs who eat the sugary, high-sucrose soy? That's right, "those animals consume more feed and grow faster."

Okay, I guess I can see why it would be good to plump up *pigs* on high-sucrose soy. But what happens when *we* eat high-sucrose soy? Won't we keep eating and gain weight, too?

I haven't been able to find an answer to that question. But it does make me wonder about the role soy may be playing in our current obesity epidemic.

Now at this point you may be thinking, "Fine, but no one in our family eats tofu, and we don't drink soy milk. So if the new high-sucrose soy is more fattening than the traditional kind, why should we care?"

Well, actually, if anyone in your family eats any kind of processed food—cereals, cookies, cakes, chips, crackers, muffins, mac 'n' cheese, goldfish crackers, chicken nuggets—you do need to be concerned. Because in the words of a 2006 article on www.gmo-compass.org, a non-profit Web site that highlights the work of independent science journalists and provides information on genetically engineered crops, "Soy Is Everywhere."

Now that's a pretty big claim, but it's no exaggeration. According to the Web site, "soy plays at least a small part in 20,000 to 30,000 products that are on the market today, whether directly as an ingredient or indirectly as a feed or nutrient source." On top of that, according to the FDA, soy is used to make soy lecithin, a "food ingredient used as an emulsifier, stabilizer, dispersing aid, and an incidental additive, such as a release agent for baked goods." In other words, soy is so useful in processed foods—helping to give those foods the consistency and shelf life they need in order to be widely distributed—that, from a manufacturer's point of view, there are good reasons for it to be "everywhere."

How had I not known this? As I began to read the labels of the processed food in my kitchen, I learned that soy was in almost everything in my cupboard. Here's just a brief list of some of the ways you and your family might be consuming soy—knowingly or, if you're like me, unknowingly:

- Margarine, vegetable oils, and mayonnaise often include soy oil.
- Chocolate desserts and baked goods often contain lecithin that has been taken from soy oil.
- Fatty foods, fortified vitamins, and even sunscreens and lotions frequently contain either tocopherol or vitamin E, which are both produced as a by-product of plant oil. (Although we don't eat sunscreens and lotions, there is some evidence that absorbing soy proteins through the skin might affect some of us, especially those of us with soy or peanut allergies.)
- Soy protein additives and soy isolate are often contained in prepared soups, sauces, meat substitutes, diet foods, and imitation milk products, such as nondairy creamer.

- Soy meal may be found in breads, snack foods, and pasta.
- Hydrolized soy protein is used in soy sauce and other seasonings.
- Soy can also be found in MSG, which is often added as a seasoning to processed and preserved foods and whose increased consumption has been linked to increased body weight.

Between the soy I ate on purpose and the soy I ate by accident, I could only imagine the havoc I had wreaked on my digestion and my metabolism—not to mention the effects I must have had on my kids' prenatal health. My Mama Guilt was growing to epic proportions, though I had to keep reminding myself that I had done the best I could with what I knew at the time.

But again, the bad news just kept coming. Because now I was about to find out that there was one more way in which our nation's kids were being loaded up with soy. Many of them had, as infants, been given soy formula. And this, I discovered, might be the most dangerous product of all.

The Littlest Victims: Soy and Infant Formula

Around the same time that the two scientists at the FDA were trying to sound the alarms about the risks of soy, other scientists were expressing concern about soy in infant formula. A 1997 study published in Britain's most prestigious medical journal, *The Lancet,* showed that infants given soy formula had in their blood serum extremely high levels of isoflavones (remember the double-edged estrogen sword?)—from five to ten times higher than women who were taking soy supplements for their menstrual cycle disturbances.

Think about that for a minute. Infants being fed on soy formula had up to ten times higher blood levels of isoflavones than adult women who were taking soy as medicine.

As we've seen, isoflavones help produce estrogen and might be toxic to the thyroid. If soy formula was loading our kids up with isoflavones, it had to be boosting their estrogen production. What effect might that be having?

Among girls and women, high levels of estrogen have been associated with breast cancer, reproductive cancers, weight gain, obesity, and early puberty. And when males are overexposed to estrogen, they may suffer from fertility problems, undescended testicles, and testicular or prostate cancer.

The *Lancet* study was cited, in fact, by Sheehan and Doerge in their 1998 warning letter to the FDA. Sheehan later said that soy-fed babies were taking part in "a large, uncontrolled and basically unmonitored human infant experiment."

But for some reason, the major governmental U.S. agency charged with protecting the health of our food did absolutely nothing about it. When I learned this, I wondered why not, especially when I found out that the British medical establishment *has* responded to the concern. Both the United Kingdom's chief medical officer and the British Dietetic Association have warned parents and pediatricians that soy formula is an absolute last resort.

Soy formula as a "last resort"? This sounded rather dire. What were other countries saying?

They, too, have expressed concern. Back in 1998, the chief advisor on Child and Youth Health of the New Zealand Ministry of Health pointed out that "[s]oy protein is a potential allergen in its own right," adding that "the use of soy formula may not be without side-effects. There is some evidence that soy formula may impair immunity and the long-term effects of contaminants of soy (e.g., aluminium and phytoestrogens) are unknown."

More recent health warnings have appeared around the globe. In 2005, the Israeli Health Ministry advised against babies receiving soy formula. The ministry also warned parents to limit the soy intake of their children under the age of eighteen: They recommended that soy in any form should be consumed no more than once a day, up to a maximum of three times a week. Adults should likewise be cautious because of soy's possible boost to breast-cancer risk among women and testicular problems among men.

In 2006, the French Food Agency announced new regulations for soy formula safety. Manufacturers are now also required to put warning labels on soy foods and soy milk, explaining that soy poses special risks to children under the age of three, children treated for thyroid disease, and women who suffer from or have a family history of breast cancer.

In November 2007, the Germans followed suit. The Federal Institute for Risk Assessment warned that soy infant formula should be given to babies only when absolutely necessary, under strict medical supervision. In December they added that soy isoflavones offer no proven health benefits while potentially posing health risks.

But our own FDA has been silent—except, of course, when it was promoting soy back in 2000. Luckily, a Web site by the prestigious pediatrician Dr. William Sears, best-selling author of *The Baby Book, The Pregnancy Book,* and many other child-care books, warns of the dangers of soy formula, even while pointing out that some 25 percent of formula-fed U.S. babies are currently consuming it.

Now this got my attention, as I had used so many of Dr. Sears's books during my first few years of motherhood, and I knew how beloved and well respected he was. If *he* thought soy was dangerous, I didn't see who could argue with him.

"There is no precedent in nature for feeding young mammals a plant-based protein," Dr. Sears points out. "Even though current biochemical knowledge has fixed some of the previous problems with soy protein for babies, we are still tampering with Mother Nature's recipe, leading us to conclude that feeding soy protein to growing babies is still experimental."

The idea of 25 percent of all formula-fed babies being part of some giant science experiment made me shudder—particularly when you consider that it's a science experiment that neither they nor their parents ever knowingly signed up for. And why wasn't our government protecting our babies the way government agencies around the world were protecting theirs?

Thank goodness for Dr. Sears. But the scary part is, he doesn't stop there. His warning includes several closely written pages about the dangers with soy formula. If you want to read the whole list of horrors, check out his Web site at www.askDrSears.com. I'll just point out two of his key concerns:

1. *As we've already seen, soy contains compounds called phytates that can deter the absorption of minerals. Since the phytate in soy binds to calcium, phosphorus, iron, and zinc, these minerals are not absorbed.* True, some companies supplement their formula with extra doses of these minerals—but some do not, which means that our babies may be missing out on vital nutritional building blocks.

And though Dr. Sears doesn't mention this, I have to wonder: What effect does it have on infant digestion to be subjected to a binding process that messes with their ability to digest proteins? Wouldn't it be better to give them something they *can* digest?

2. *Giving infants soy formula potentially puts them at greater risk for allergies.* This is such an important point that you should read it in Dr. Sears's own words: "Giving an infant soy in the early months before intestinal closure may predispose the infant to soy allergies later on. Since soy is used as a filler in so many foods in the American diet, this is a serious concern."

"A serious concern" is putting it mildly! By the time I read those words, I was jumping out of my seat. Thankfully, I had no Mama Guilt over soy formula: my children had all been given regular cow's milk formula after I had stopped nursing them. But what about all the mothers who thought soy was safe? And there were more than a few of us out there. According to a May 2008 report from the American Academy of Pediatrics (AAP), "Soy protein–based formulas in the United States may account for nearly 20% to 25% of the formula market."

Meanwhile, given all the soy I'd eaten during pregnancy and while breast-feeding, I could empathize with the feelings of parents who might come upon Dr. Sears's warnings too late. And I wondered why, if we'd known about these dangers since the 1997 *Lancet* study, our soy formula wasn't labeled as potentially hazardous to infants and why our medical establishment and government agencies weren't leaping to protect nursing mothers and their infants, as their counterparts were doing in Europe and New Zealand.

Later, I would wonder whether the influence of the multibillion-dollar soybean industry had anything to do with the unwillingness of our doctors and government agencies to do what the Australians, British, Israelis, Germans, French, and New Zealanders have done. I would start looking more closely at the ties between the agricultural and chemical companies and the medical establishment, and I'd see new meaning in the fact that some of the doctors on FAAN's medical board had been associated with an enormous chemical corporation called Monsanto, which just happened to be responsible for producing over 80 percent of the world's soy in the form of a widely used genetically engineered soybean.

But I hadn't quite gotten there yet. First, I was preoccupied with Dr. Sears's reference to soy allergies, which reminded me of the questions I'd started asking when I read that first press release about "the potential of genetically engineered foods to cause allergic reactions." As I'd reasoned, both soy and peanuts were legumes. Could children's consumption of soy formula be in any way related to the rise of the peanut allergy?

The Allergy Detective Investigates Soy

Scientists have a fancy name for what happens when a person's allergies to one food seem to set off an allergy to another. They call it *cross-reactivity*. Often, when two substances are similar, an allergy to one predicts an allergy to the other. Since peanuts and soy share similar protein structures, many people who are allergic to one food may also be allergic to the other.

Cross-reactivity produced tragic results for several children in Sweden, who died quite suddenly from anaphylactic shock after eating foods that contained soy. These children were known to be allergic to peanuts. But since their parents had never been warned about potential links between legumes, the families had no idea that soy, too, might trigger a deadly response.

When I first learned about cross-reactivity, I started searching for scientific papers about the condition. To my surprise, I found many, including one with three authors—Scott Sicherer, Hugh Sampson, and A. Wesley Burks. Do those names ring any bells with you? They did with me: all three physicians are on the medical board of FAAN. Now it seemed that two of them—Hugh Sampson and Wesley Burks—were actually trying to create genetically engineered foods. As we saw in chapter 2, they were both working with the Peanut Genome Initiative, trying to develop a nonallergenic peanut. And as we also saw, Dr. Sampson helped invent a genetically engineered protein for the Monsanto Corporation.

The doctors' article is known as a "review article," that is, a review of all the scientific literature on a particular topic. In this case, the doctors were reviewing the relationship between allergies to peanuts and allergies to soy.

My jaw kept dropping as I read through their work, thinking of how naïve I'd been. Because I had found none of this information on the FAAN Web site, I had assumed no one associated with that group was aware of it. But here were three members of FAAN's medical board frankly discussing the issue. They cited all the evidence that many people are indeed allergic to both peanuts and soy. They acknowledged that a peanut-allergic person might react to the soy protein, and vice versa. They even explained the science behind the connection, pointing out that "peanut-allergic individuals had extensive IgE binding to other legumes, including soy."

In other words, those potent IgE antibodies—the ones that attack the toxic invaders and might cause hives, redness, swelling, or anaphylactic shock—weren't only triggered by peanuts. Those antibodies—though originally intended only to attack peanuts—might accidentally be sent flooding into the body at the tiniest hint of soy.

Wasn't this exactly what had happened to those children in Sweden? Shouldn't parents of peanut-allergic kids be warned that soy, too, might trigger an attack? Especially given the sudden increases that we are seeing in the number of children with peanut allergy?

But, at the end of their review, Sampson and his colleagues basically conclude that given how few children have peanut allergy, we shouldn't worry about the cross-reactivity between peanut and soy allergies. And since the review was conducted in 2000, maybe back then they were right.

But since we've seen a 20 percent annual increase in the number of children with peanut allergy over the last several years, wouldn't it make sense to conduct another review?

Of course, as we've seen, soy is in *everything* these days: processed foods, salad dressings, fast-food burgers, even vitamins. And, as I've understood the research, most peanut-allergic kids *don't* seem to have unhealthy responses to soy. I can see why physicians and scientists would be unwilling to recommend that parents restrict their kids' diets needlessly, fearful of an allergic reaction that may never come to pass. It's hard enough keeping kids away from peanuts—why stop them from eating soy, too, if it's not necessary?

Not surprisingly, this was the reaction of FAAN and its medical board. After I posted information in an AllergyKids newsletter and on the AllergyKids blog about the Swedish children and the possibility of soy-peanut cross-reactivity, parents became concerned, and naturally, they turned to FAAN for a second opinion.

Well, to put it bluntly, FAAN went wild. They even quoted my citation of Ingrid Yman, PhD, of the Swedish National Food Administration: "If your child is allergic to peanuts, you should consider eliminating soy as well as all peanuts from your child's diet, even if your child has never reacted poorly to soy in the past." As it happens, my article had included a couple more sentences from Dr. Yman that FAAN chose not to quote. Her words were based on the tragic deaths of the Swedish children: "Some sensitive children have 'hidden' soy allergies that manifest for the first time with a severe—even fatal—reaction to even the low levels of 'hidden' soy commonly found in processed food products. Those at the highest risk suffer from asthma as well as peanut allergy."

Having quoted the first part of Dr. Yman's statement, the FAAN Web site went on to refute it. They basically told parents not to worry about cross-reactivity, especially because restricting soy in their children's diets might cause nutritional problems. They pointed out that soy is used extensively in Asian countries, yet peanut allergies in Asia are rare. They also asserted—correctly, of course—that most people with peanut allergies have no problem eating soy. Finally, they cited a 2005 Finnish study published in the journal *Pediatric Allergy and Immunology* that supposedly refutes the idea of cross-reactivity. In that study, researchers concluded that for infants diagnosed with milk allergy, exposure to soy formula during the first two years of life did not increase the risk of developing a peanut allergy.

But why had FAAN disclosed the soy-peanut link only after I had highlighted it? Didn't parents deserve to know about the risks that soy might present to their peanut-allergic children?

Of course, I can see both sides. I read the Finnish study, and it makes sense to me. And I can see that parents whose kids are allergic to peanuts shouldn't have to worry unduly about protecting their kids from soy. If most peanut-allergic kids can tolerate soy, why make them and their parents crazy trying to avoid it?

On the other hand, a simple warning of the potential cross-reactivity allows parents to make an informed choice when it comes to feeding their kids soy. FAAN's failure to warn us of this potential risk strikes me as slightly irresponsible, not to say condescending, especially since some research suggests that there really *is* a risk.

Consider, for example, a 1999 U.S. study that, like the Finnish study, focused on children with cow's milk allergies. Coauthored by FAAN's own physicians—Hugh Sampson, Allan Bock, and Robert Zeiger—this study found that sensitization to soy was reported in 10 percent to 14 percent of infants with cow's milk allergy.

When I first read about these studies, I was confused. Why were they focusing on kids with cow's milk allergies? Then I realized that these dairy-allergic kids are precisely the ones who are most likely to be given soy formula, as an alternative to milk-based formulas. But if a significant percent of these milk-allergic kids are also allergic to soy, they *shouldn't* be given soy formula. In fact, that was the basis for the American Academy of Pediatrics's 2008 recommendation that soy formula be prescribed cautiously, if at all: "although most infants with IgE-mediated cow milk [*sic*] allergy will tolerate soy formula, because of the 10% to 14% cross-over rate, the use of an extensively hydrolyzed protein formula rather than a soy formula may be considered in infants allergic to cow milk formula." In other words, even if your kids *are* allergic to milk, they may be better off with an "extensively hydrolyzed protein formula" rather than with soy, just in case they're among the 10 to 14 percent of children with milk allergies who are *also* allergic to soy.

When I read that this was the position of the American Academy of Pediatrics (AAP), I had to wonder why it wasn't also FAAN's position, especially since members of FAAN's medical board were involved in some of the research on which the AAP based its recommendation. FAAN itself has said that they don't want to worry parents unduly, and that they don't want to needlessly deprive kids of the potential nutritional benefits of soy. But given FAAN's previous acceptance of funds from processed-food companies—which, as we've seen, rely heavily on soy—I had to wonder if there were other reasons FAAN was downplaying these concerns.

Meanwhile, what about the research that goes even further—suggesting not only that some kids have multiple allergies but also that early exposure to soy might actually help *create* a peanut allergy? For example, a 2003 British study conducted by Gideon Lack of St. Mary's Hospital at Imperial College in London followed almost 14,000 children from the womb through age six—a far bigger and more comprehensive study than the others we've reviewed, and one that included *all* types of children, not just those allergic to cow's milk.

The British study turned up a shocking fact: Kids who had been given soy formula as infants seemed almost three times as likely to develop a peanut allergy later on. Only 8.3 percent of *all* the kids in the study had been given soy formula—but 24.5 percent of the peanut-allergic kids had had it. And, the researchers pointed out, "of the 10 children for whom data on the first consumption of soy milk or soy formula were available, 9 had consumed soy before reacting to peanuts."

Could this be why peanut allergies were appearing in children at younger ages? It sure *looked* like soy formula was triggering a peanut allergy.

The British study made some other connections as well. Apparently some infants had developed peanut allergies from the skin creams and oils that their mothers had rubbed them with—moisturizers that contained, you guessed it, peanut oil. Sometimes the moms were trying to treat diaper rash, and sometimes they were applying creams to their children's scaly scalps. Either way, kids who'd been treated with peanut-oil products were 6.8 times more likely to develop peanut allergies, according to a report in the March 2003 *New England Journal of Medicine*.

The previous year, a Wisconsin doctor made a similar connection. According to a 2002 report published by a local Wisconsin TV station, Dr. Paul Kuwayama had become curious about the link between his patients' peanut allergies and their consumption of infant soy formula. When he looked at his patients' records, he found that some 62 percent of his peanut-allergic patients had once been fed on soy formula.

I hate to quote one lone Wisconsin doctor's statistics when I could be citing a major study. The problem is, there don't seem to be many major studies. As with food allergies in general, the research just isn't being done, despite the fact that, as we've seen, the peanut allergy appears to be increasing at a rate of 20 percent a year.

So I get that scientists are divided on this topic—though the British study of almost 14,000 kids seems a lot bigger and more reliable than any of the others. To me, that *is* a definitive study, and the British medical establishment and government health agencies have taken it as such. Based on that and other research, they've gone on to warn parents about the dangers of soy, so that parents can make an informed choice when it comes to protecting their infants. So why hasn't the same thing happened here in the United States? And why is FAAN so defensive about this?

When you look at the behavior of the scientists and physicians over the past twenty years, a suggestive picture emerges. When the potential for the allergenicity of soy was first raised in the 1990s, many prominent scientists were part of the investigation of this crucial health issue. But then, a funny thing happened. Many of them either distanced themselves from food allergy groups, as did Dr. Fred McDaniel Atkins, or took funding from food corporations, as did Drs. Burks and Sampson. But none of them offered definitive refutations of the concerns they and their colleagues had raised. Whether that's because they had changed their minds or changed their loyalties, I have no way of knowing.

But I have to say it: The failure to fully disclose all relevant information here in the United States is one of the most crazy-making parts of this whole issue. Even if we don't know which study is correct, shouldn't we at least know about the debate? Shouldn't every parent whose kid has a peanut allergy know that some children, at least, have died from what sure *looks* like a cross-reactive allergic response? Shouldn't the CDC at least be tracking food allergy deaths, especially if one of the few studies that the CDC has conducted in the last few years showed a 265 percent increase in hospitalizations related to food allergic reactions? Shouldn't soy formula at least be labeled, as it is abroad, with warnings of its possible adverse effects on our infants given that even the American Academy of Pediatrics says an "additional study is warranted"? You seriously have to wonder why we haven't valued the lives of our babies the way the lives of children around the world have been valued.

More important, can we trust the word of physicians who are receiving funds from the peanut and soybean industries? Can we trust a nonprofit that puts those physicians on its medical board or that takes money from a processed-food manufacturer to fund its Web site without disclosing these ties? Don't the peanut, soybean, and processed-food industries have a vested interest in presenting a particular point of view, one that reassures us about the safety of soybeans (found in so many processed foods) and the limited nature of peanut allergies? Why have other developed countries warned parents about the dangers of soy, while our government agencies refuse to listen even to their own scientists?

Does it have anything to do with the fact that the United States has the world's largest soybean industry?

Call me cynical, but I couldn't help thinking that corporate financial interests are involved. The theme song to Donald Trump's television series *The Apprentice,* the O'Jays' "For the Love of Money," ran through my head: *"Money, money, money, mo-ney!"* A few months later, I'd learn that the links among the science and medical communities, U.S. corporations, and the U.S. government were closer than I'd ever suspected.

Meanwhile, though, I was still obsessed with understanding the science behind all of the recent changes in soy. And the next science I looked into seemed to me the stuff of nightmares—taken straight from a science fiction movie—the world of biotechnology and the genetic manipulation of our food.

The Allergy Detective Looks at Genetically Modified Soy

I must admit to an intense fascination with the whole world of genetic engineering. It scares me, it baffles me, and sometimes it outrages me—but it never fails to interest me. I guess that's a good thing, because I do think that understanding this major new development in how we grow and consume food is crucial for every one of us.

I also have to admit that the whole premise sounds so science fiction–like to me, I have a hard time grasping that it's real. I still can't wrap my mind around the discovery that corporations have been manipulating our food supply this way since the mid-1990s, especially since I never had any idea that this was going on.

I had no idea, for example, that according to the U.S. Department of Agriculture, 92 percent of soy grown worldwide is genetically modified, as is 80 percent of the corn, not to mention 86 percent of all U.S. cotton. According to Cornell University, there are twelve genetically engineered (GE) plant species that have been approved for commercial production in the United States: corn, cotton, potatoes, tomatoes, soybeans, canola, sugar beets, rice, flax, squash/zucchini, papaya, and chicory (radicchio). But whether or not our minds can take in those facts, our bodies are already taking in that food.

So welcome to our brave new world! From here through chapter 5, I'll break it all down for you, as simply as possible, so that by the time you're done, you'll know what you need to know to make your own reasoned, informed decision about this fascinating topic.

Scrambled Genes

On the simplest level, genetic engineering involves manipulating genes, altering an organism's DNA to create a new trait. A genetically modified crop might be developed to resist bugs, for example, or to withstand frequent spraying with herbicides.

In fact, that was the inspiration for genetically modified soy. Monsanto, a giant biotech and chemical company, was already making Roundup, an herbicide that is great at killing weeds—but that also kills crops. So in 1996, Monsanto began to market Roundup Ready soybeans, which were genetically engineered to withstand megadoses of Roundup. Farmers who plant this new form of soybean can spray their crops as often as they like. While weeds are blasted into oblivion, the soy plants continue to flourish.

Even in the mid-1990s, people knew that genetic engineering held some potential hazards. In fact, even some executives at Monsanto were raising serious concerns.

For example, an article in *Consumers' Research Magazine* quotes James D. Astwood, manager of Monsanto's Protein Characterization and Safety Center, as he spoke at a food allergy conference in 1994. Anticipating many of the later objections to genetically modified foods, Astwood acknowledged that mixing the DNA from two separate plants might transfer allergens along with the genes.

"[I]magine if you moved an allergen from peanuts into corn or into wheat," he said. "A peanut-allergic person knows how to avoid peanuts, but would [he] know to avoid wheat? The answer is no."

However, Astwood said, Monsanto was committed to developing new ways "to predict the allergenic potential of new products." As we'll soon see, the company never did manage to do this, but in 1994, it certainly sounded like a responsible corporate citizen. And even its own scientists thought that their new genetically modified crops *might* trigger new allergies, simply by making potential allergens more widespread.

Remember, soy is *everywhere*. It's in almost every kind of processed food, in soy-based infant formula, and in many conventional formulas as well. So if genetically modified soy contained an extra allergen, picked up from the genetic material of some other plant, that could play havoc with the immune system of all the millions of people—and infants—who consume soy.

Astwood's concern seemed validated in 1996, when University of Nebraska researchers discovered just the type of cross-allergenic incident that he had described. The Nebraska scientists found that genetically modified soybeans had been altered by the addition of proteins from the Brazil nut.

As you recall from chapter 1, proteins are what an allergic person reacts to. "Toxic invader" proteins trigger the IgE or IgG molecules, which then flood the body with the cytokines and histamines of an allergic attack. Since the Brazil nut protein had been engineered into the soy, if you were allergic to Brazil nuts, you would have reacted badly to any food that contained the genetically modified soy—without ever realizing that it was the hidden Brazil nut gene, not the soy itself, that had triggered the response.

The Brazil-nutty soy never made it onto the market. But if it had, its label would have been misleading. That's because U.S. government regulations don't require identifying food as "genetically modified," giving a whole new meaning to the phrase "Let the buyer beware!"

A few years later, U.K. scientists also sounded the alarm. A March 12, 1999, article in the *Daily Express* revealed that in a single year, health complaints caused by soy—at the time, the predominant genetically modified food—had risen by 50 percent.

According to the article, "Researchers at the York Nutritional Laboratory said their findings provide real evidence that GM food could have a tangible, harmful impact on the human body." Symptoms associated with soy included chronic fatigue syndrome, irritable bowel syndrome, and other digestion problems, as well as headache, lethargy, acne, and eczema.

As we've seen, these responses might well be allergic reactions. And indeed, for the first time in seventeen years of testing, soy had made the top-ten list of U.K. allergic complaints.

The debates over GM soy continued. A new chapter was written on August 13, 2002, at a meeting of the Food Biotechnology Subcommittee of the Food Advisory Committee, a multiagency committee that included representatives from the Department of Health and Human Services and the Center for Food Safety and Applied Nutrition, a division of the FDA. This government-sponsored meeting involved a wide range of participants: scientists, government officials, industry representatives, and private physicians, including former FAAN board member Fred McDaniel Atkins, MD, and Monsanto safety officer James Astwood. The committee's task was to discuss the potential allergenicity of genetically engineered foods.

If you follow the minutes of this contentious meeting, you can see how hotly debated the topic was, and how high tempers rose. You also get a sense of how new the issues were, even in 2002, and how uncertain even these top-level scientists and officials were about how to evaluate them.

The committee's acting chair was Edward N. Brandt, Jr., MD, PhD, nominated by President Ronald Reagan in 1981 to serve as assistant secretary in the U.S. Department of Health and Human Services, as well as a former U.S. representative to the World Health Organization's executive board. In response to a discussion on the safety of genetically engineered foods, Brandt actually said, "Of course, we [haven't] . . . worked into this some kind of a test for allergenicity, per se."

A swift reply came from Dean Metcalfe, the government scientist who headed the National Institutes of Health's Laboratory of Allergic Diseases and who served as director of the Allergy and Immunology Training Program at the National Institutes of Health's National Institute of Allergy and Infectious Diseases. Metcalfe explained that although you could test genetically engineered crops for *known* proteins, it was the unintended creation of *new* proteins that made it difficult to test GM crops for allergenicity. Creating new proteins was what genetic engineering was all about—and since these proteins had never before existed, how did you find out whether people might be allergic to them?

When I read Metcalfe's remarks, I thought, *Wait a minute. These guys are straight-out admitting that genetically engineered crops might be producing brand-new allergens.*

But how could industry have introduced these crops into the food supply if they had no test to make sure that they *weren't* going to spark new allergies? How could the U.S. government have allowed our corporations to do something so risky?

Remember, even Monsanto's James Astwood had raised this possibility as early as 1994. Why hadn't anyone done something back then? And if not then, why not in 2002?

I looked at the minutes of that government-sponsored meeting and all I could see was that neither industry nor government nor private physicians were doing *anything*. No one was insisting that these potentially allergenic crops be withdrawn until they *could* be properly tested. No one was pointing out that the number of allergic kids had already started to rise. How many more kids would have to develop allergies before someone got upset about this?

FAAN's former medical director said it best. "To me," Dr. Atkins commented, "the logical problem is we are going to take that stuff and feed it to the public without [their] informed consent."

Yes, sir, Dr. Atkins. That *is* a problem—a very big problem. And you know what? Here we are, seven years later—and the public is still eating "that stuff."

Genetically Modified Soy: What's the Evidence?

Okay. So we know that in 1994, 1996, and 2002, U.S. and U.K. scientists were raising concerns about genetically modified soy and allergies. But what else do we know about genetically modified soy? What can science tell us about how this new food affects us?

Well, precious little, as it turns out. Of the studies that have been done on genetically modified soy, only one has been done using humans, rather than animals, in its research.

That one human study, though, is extremely disturbing. A July 27, 2004, report from the U.S. National Academy of Sciences says that parts of the altered gene in genetically modified soy were transferred into the DNA of the bacteria that live in the human gut. If these altered genes were not eliminated along with other waste products—as genetic engineers had assumed—but rather went on to live in our gut bacteria, they might change our immune and intestinal systems in unpredictable ways, thereby compromising our immune systems.

As disturbing as that human study may be, I'm even more troubled by a 2005 animal study conducted at the Russian Academy of Sciences. Dr. Irina Ermakova discovered that more than half the offspring (55.6 percent) of rats fed on genetically modified soy died in the first three weeks of life—*six to eight times as many* as those born to mothers given either conventional soy (9 percent) or no soy (6.8 percent). Six times as many rat babies (36 percent) were severely underweight as well, compared to those in the other groups (6 percent).

Several other European studies suggest the dangers of genetically modified soy. Italian research, for example, showed that genetically modified soy affected the liver and pancreas in mice. In Australia, researchers discovered that genetically modified peas caused lung damage. And a May 2005 article in the London-based *Independent* told of a "secret report" prepared by Monsanto showing that rats who ate genetically modified corn had smaller kidneys and higher blood counts than other rats, suggesting that their immune systems might have been damaged.

A secret report? Why wasn't Monsanto coming forward and making this study public? Could it be that since the company is also the global leader in the production of genetically modified corn, it wanted to protect its product?

Coming to Terms with Genetically Modified Soy

Perhaps the introduction of genetically modified soy has nothing to do with the allergy epidemic—though in my opinion, that possibility is highly unlikely. But even if genetically modified soy isn't making kids more allergic, why aren't we more concerned with its health risks the way other developed countries are? Why aren't we demanding that the companies who make this product must also take the extra precaution of proving that it's safe before we and our children consume it? Why aren't we following the lead of consumers in Europe, England, Australia, and Japan, and insisting that genetically modified ingredients be clearly identified on food labels, so that we at least have the option of making an informed choice?

When I read Dr. Ermakova's study, all I could think of was how many times I had reached for the soybeans during my four pregnancies. How many times I had exposed my unborn children to the risks that had caused a six- to eightfold increase in infant deaths among Dr. Ermakova's baby rats. How many times I had risked flooding my kids' immune systems with brand-new proteins whose effects had never been tested on humans—because they'd never before existed.

The thing that's so upsetting is, I didn't have a choice. I didn't know that soy was genetically modified. I didn't know that genetically modified soy had been linked to increased incidence of allergies. I didn't know that the companies who made genetically modified soy and the government agencies who were supposed to regulate it had discussed, well before my first pregnancy, the possibility that this new product might make people—including my children!—more allergic. I didn't even know that I *was* eating genetically modified soy—because the packages were never labeled.

My rational side said, *Robyn, you did the best you could.* But my Mommy Mind-set said, *Serve up another helping of Mama Guilt.*

What the hell. At this point, it tasted better than soy.

4

MILK MONEY

Despite the guilt and anguish that I felt when I thought about the dangers of GM soy, I also felt relieved. I honestly thought this might be the key to the mystery that all of us in the allergy community had been trying to solve, and that all I had to do was get the right people to listen to my theories.

Now, I can't believe how naïve I was. How could I have thought that so many doctors, researchers, and scientists had never even noticed the connection between the allergy epidemic and GM foods, especially when my own introduction to it had come through a press release announcing a new study at a major university? But since none of the FAAN members I knew was talking about it, and since the information wasn't on FAAN's Web site, I simply assumed that nobody knew.

So yes, I was just exactly that naïve. And maybe that was a good thing in the end, since my naïveté led me to reach out to other allergy parents trying to spread the word.

I began by sending an e-mail to an allergy mom I knew in New York, someone who raised lots of money for the cause and had told me of her connection with FAAN medical board member Hugh Sampson, MD, one of the most respected allergy experts in the country. I asked her to ask Dr. Sampson about my theory and find out what he thought about it.

She did—but he just didn't seem interested. Basically, he told her that there were lots of theories out there, and this seemed like just one more.

I couldn't understand his response. If the doctor had explained why there was no connection between genetic engineering and allergies, I would have been happy to listen to his reasoning. But he seemed to be dismissing a potentially powerful explanation, as if we shouldn't be worrying our pretty little heads about this.

Perhaps I'm being unfair, because this woman was satisfied with Dr. Sampson's answer—but I wasn't. And now, of course, it appears that Dr. Sampson knew better. He had been part of a 2001 Department of Health and Human Services workshop called Assessment of the Allergenic Potential of Genetically Modified Foods. He had coauthored the review article with two other FAAN board members on the cross-reactivity of peanuts and soy. He had even helped investigate the very first big GM-related scandal, when the genetically engineered StarLink corn accidentally entered the food supply in 2001 and seemed to provoke a series of dangerous allergic reactions. (I'll explain that incident in detail in chapter 5.) If he knew all that, why wasn't a full explanation of the controversy, along with his reasons for no longer being concerned, laid out on the FAAN Web site? In fact, Dr. Sampson has never publicly explained why, despite his involvement in the StarLink investigation, he now believes we need not be concerned about the potential allergenicity of genetically modified foods.

Call it Mama Bear instinct, call it Research Wonk stubbornness, call it whatever you like. Because although one of the most respected experts in the country had told me to forget it, I just couldn't let go of this new idea. I felt I couldn't approach FAAN directly—after all, our legal tussle had taken place only a few months earlier. But I thought that if I could just find the facts and figures to back up my position, maybe someone would listen.

So back I went to my computer, looking for answers and discovering new questions. And this time, they led me to milk.

Falling Through the Looking Glass

Every time I look into genetic engineering, one name keeps coming up: Monsanto. This giant agrichemical corporation was the pioneering force behind DDT, Agent Orange, genetically modified soy, and aspartame (a.k.a. NutraSweet and Equal). At the time I began researching Monsanto in 2006, it was a $30 billion agrichemical corporation that appeared to have at least one of their products in every home in America. As of this writing, in the summer of 2008, the company is worth more than $72 billion.

If you've never heard of Monsanto, you're not alone: before 2006, I hadn't either. So let me introduce you. Monsanto is a chemical company that was initially known for its global dominance in the pesticide market. As an early pioneer in the growing field of genetic engineering, Monsanto now owns 90 percent of the U.S. soy market in the form of its genetically modified Roundup Ready soy. In fact, Monsanto is responsible for much of the food we eat: it makes the genetically altered corn seeds that dominate the market, and it's also the creator of genetically engineered potatoes, pigs, and other increasingly common foods. In addition, the company produces safety glass, dishwasher detergent, vinyl siding, and the fibers that go into Astroturf, as well as many other chemical and manufactured products. And its corn can be used for ethanol.

Once I started looking into the company, I couldn't believe what a powerful political and economic force it is. As I've said, I was raised in a conservative southern family and I have always loved my country. But I'll be honest: what I learned about Monsanto really shook my faith there for a while. As I read about how much control Monsanto had over our food supply, our farmers, and, apparently, our government, I felt as though I had just fallen through Alice's looking glass. How could one company have so much power?

I never expected to learn that the government and the system I'd always supported could have such an intimate relationship with such a powerful company—and, I would later discover, such a greedy one. Yet the story seemed to start innocently enough—with a simple glass of plain white milk.

Raging Hormones

For the past fifteen years, much of our nation's milk has come from cows injected with a genetically engineered growth hormone. That hormone has two interchangeable names: recombinant bovine somatotrophine (rBST) and recombinant bovine growth hormone (rBGH).

RBGH has dominated the milk market almost since the FDA approved it in 1993. It's made by only a single company, Monsanto, which markets it under the trademarked name Posilac. As the inventor and patent-holder of this genetically engineered hormone, Monsanto is the only company allowed to sell it, enjoying a complete monopoly on the drug. (At least, that was the situation until Monsanto sold their Posilac division to Elanco, a division of Eli Lilly, in October 2008.)

Still, Posilac was the first genetically engineered product that Monsanto brought to market, and they promoted it heavily for fourteen years. Today the Associated Press (AP), the New York Times, and the rest of the media have called Posilac "controversial" (the AP headline actually referred to it as "a bumper crop of controversy"), and the company is disassociating itself from the product. But the story of what Monsanto did to promote Posilac serves as a disturbing lesson in the politics of food.

So what is rBGH anyway? Although the product is made in a lab, it's designed to mimic a hormone that's naturally produced in a cow's pituitary glands. It's injected into cows every two weeks to boost their hormonal activity, causing them to produce an additional 10 to 15 percent more milk, or about one extra gallon each day.

As of 1998, about one-third of the nation's cows were in herds being treated with this growth hormone. Monsanto biotechnology communications director Gary Barton adds that "because milk from many dairies is mixed together, essentially *all* . . . milk is treated [with rBGH]," except of course milk that's specifically labeled as rBGH- or rBST-free, or milk labeled "organic" (emphasis added).

If all you knew about rBGH and this hormone was that it increased milk production, you might think it was a good thing. Why shouldn't we use every means at our disposal to boost the supply of such a nutritious food? Why shouldn't farmers make more profit on each dairy cow they own? And why shouldn't consumers welcome additional gallons of milk, since that would seem likely to lower milk prices?

Well, besides increasing milk production, rBGH apparently does a few other things, too.

First of all, the product seems to be hazardous to the cows. The package itself warns of such bovine problems as "increases in cystic ovaries and disorders of the uterus," "decreases in gestation length and birthweight of calves," and "increased risk of clinical mastitis." Mastitis is a painful type of udder infection that causes cows to pump out bacteria and pus along with milk (women can get it while nursing), requiring treatment with antibiotics and other meds that can end up in the milk.

When I first read this, I had to stop and walk away from the computer for a few minutes. How many bottles and sippy cups had I filled with milk? Why hadn't I known about rBGH when I was pouring countless bowls of cereal for my children? I shuddered at the thought that along with the milk, I had also been giving them doses of growth hormone and antibiotics, not to mention potentially exposing them to cow bacteria and udder pus.

As we saw in chapter 2, overexposure to antibiotics tends to kill off the friendly bacteria in our intestines—bacteria that we need for our digestion and immune system. Many doctors believe that too many antibiotics at too early an age is part of the reason that kids are more likely to be allergic: their immune systems don't have the microbial environment that they require. Now that I know how many extra antibiotics our kids are getting in their milk, cheese, and yogurt and from our prenatal diet, I have to wonder if that's another factor in the allergy epidemic.

Remember, too, that allergies are the body's response to proteins that it considers toxic invaders, and that genetically engineered proteins may spark new allergies. According to CNN and a recent study published in the *Journal of Allergy and Immunology,* milk allergy is now the most common food allergy in the United States, having risen to the number one position in the last ten years. Might rBGH be a factor in that increase?

But let's get back to the cows, because Posilac can hurt them in several more ways. The label also warns of possible increase in digestive disorders, including diarrhea; increased numbers of lacerations on the cows' hocks (shins); and a higher rate of *subclinical* mastitis.

I'm emphasizing the word "subclinical" because I find the idea so disturbing. Bad enough when dairy cows get visibly sick, because then they're treated with antibiotics that end up in our milk. But what about the cows who are getting sick at a subclinical level—a level so subtle that farmers don't notice it? Think of the bacteria and pus pouring out of those inflamed udders—infections that aren't even being treated. How does drinking *that* milk affect us, our kids, and the babies in our wombs?

Those are just the problems acknowledged on the Posilac product label. Another concern is that the extra hormones drain the cows' bones of calcium, so that they tend to become lame. Monsanto has disputed this claim, but the Canadian federal health agency doesn't buy the company's arguments. Instead, it found that "the risk of clinical lameness was increased approximately 50 percent" in cows that were given rBGH. Partly as a result, Canada has prohibited the product, concluding that it "presents a sufficient and unacceptable threat to the safety of dairy cows."

Indeed, cows hopped-up on rBGH typically live for only about two years after they start receiving the drug. By contrast, cows who *aren't* injected with rBGH live on for four to ten years.

Canada isn't the only country to disallow the use of rBGH. The genetically altered hormone is not approved for use in the European Union, Japan, Australia, and New Zealand. In addition, the U.N. agency that sets food safety standards, Codex Alimentarius, has twice concluded there was no consensus on the safety of rBGH.

Farmers themselves have noticed problems with the product. In addition to the expense of the drug, rBGH results in higher feed bills, higher vet bills, and more cows removed from the herd due to illness or low productivity. One study found that 25 to 40 percent of dairy farmers who tried rBGH soon gave it up because it wasn't profitable enough to justify the damage to their cows. Other farmers have said that they see how hard the product is on cows, and they don't want to subject their animals to such treatment.

Okay, so that's how Posilac hurts cows. But I'm way more concerned about us and our kids. How does having a genetically altered hormone in our milk supply affect *us*?

Cash Cows

As you might expect, the news is not so great. First, Monsanto's product hits us in the pocketbook. Our U.S. dairy farmers already produce more milk than we can drink, so our government buys up the surplus with our taxpayer dollars. When farmers use rBGH to step up milk production, the government then has to use *more* taxpayer dollars to buy the additional milk. Otherwise, the extra milk on the market would drive the price of milk so low that many farmers would go out of business.

As a result, from 1995 to 2006, dairy program subsidies cost U.S. taxpayers $3.6 billion. More than half of that money went toward contract payments to milk farmers for lost income.

Second, there's the effect of Posilac on the smaller family farms. Since giving cows the growth hormone steps up milk production, profits flow to big dairy farmers, big dairy processors, and, of course, Monsanto. But some family farmers believe that the growth of the large dairy businesses comes at their detriment.

"More milk means fewer farmers," says John Bunting, a New York dairy farmer quoted in the *Washington Independent*. That's because the more milk that's on the market, the lower prices go, resulting in the government paying out even more subsidies. The big milk farmers get their subsidies and ride out the price wars, but the little guy, who has smaller subsidies or none at all, goes out of business.

Most worrisome of all, however, is rBGH's effect on our health. As early as 1998, an article in *The Lancet,* the prestigious British medical journal, reported that women with even relatively small increases of a hormone known as insulin-like growth factor 1 (IGF-1) were up to seven times more likely to develop premenopausal breast cancer.

And guess what? According to a January 1996 report in the *International Journal of Health Services,* rBGH milk has up to ten times the IGF-1 levels of natural milk. More recent studies have put the figure even higher, at something like twentyfold.

Now stop and think about that for a minute. Breast cancer used to be something that women got later in life. Premenopausal breast cancer was so rare that when young women presented their physicians with breast cancer symptoms, the doctors often failed to diagnose it, simply because it was so unlikely that an "older women's disease" would be found among young women.

But according to the Young Survival Coalition, one in 229 women between the ages of thirty and thirty-nine will be diagnosed with breast cancer in the next ten years. Why are all these young women now getting breast cancer? And what about the effects of IGF-1-laden milk on older women, who are already at greater risk for breast cancer?

In case you think that the rising cancer rates have something to do with genetics, stop and think again. According to the Breast Cancer Fund, one in eight women now has breast cancer. But only 10 percent of those cases can be linked to genetics. In other words, 90 percent of breast cancers being diagnosed today are being triggered by factors in our environment. Doesn't it seem logical that there might be a connection between a breast cancer–causing hormone introduced into our milk in 1994 and the increasing rates of breast cancer?

IGF-1 has also been implicated in prostate and colon cancer. An article in the *Washington Independent* quotes Kaiser Permanente internist Dr. Jenny Pompilio as saying that even "subtle amounts" of IGF-1 can increase the risk of cancer.

"It's been known for years that that particular hormone is linked with cancers [because of its effects] on the endocrine system," says Dr. Pompilio. (The endocrine system regulates the release of hormones and is instrumental in regulating metabolism, growth, development, puberty, tissue function, and also plays a role in determining mood.) As Dr. Pompilio explains, "The endocrine system is so sensitive that subtle effects can make a difference."

Now, if you're like me, your next question probably is, *So, if we know all of this, how the hell did this hormone find its way into our dairy products?* How did our government agencies, responsible for ensuring the safety of our food, allow the use of this growth hormone and the sale of IGF-1-laden milk? Why was Posilac not used in Europe, Japan, Canada, Australia, and New Zealand, but used so freely right here in the United States?

Well, Dr. Henry Miller, who was in charge of biotech issues for the FDA during the time that Monsanto's Posilac was approved, had an interesting comment on the whole area of biotechnology, a term that usually includes genetic modification and includes rBGH: "In this area," Dr. Miller said, "the U.S. government agencies have done exactly what big agribusiness has asked them to do and told them to do."

Dr. Miller's statement is supported by a 1992 FDA policy statement on genetic engineering that neatly evades any government responsibility at all. The year before the FDA approved the first genetically engineered protein, milk's rBGH, it said, "Ultimately, it is the food producer who is responsible for assuring safety."

What? The corporations are expected to police themselves? Does the FDA believe that all corporations are staffed entirely with altruistic, ethical executives whose primary concern is product safety and not profit? Or that executive compensation is tied to safety, not sales?

Sure, responsible corporations welcome government supervision because it means that everybody has to play by the same rules. But years of stock market analyses and reading the *Wall Street Journal* have taught me that it doesn't always happen this way. Haven't we learned anything from the tobacco industry?

So I wasn't surprised to learn that Monsanto, too, has a slightly different take on the issue. In an October 25, 1998, *New York Times Magazine* article by Michael Pollan, Monsanto corporate communications director Phil Angell put the responsibility for product safety squarely back on the FDA: "Monsanto should not have to vouchsafe the safety of biotech food," Angell declared. "Our interest is in selling as much of it as possible. Assuring its safety is the F.D.A.'s job."

So gentlemen, please, make up your minds. *Whose job is it to ensure food safety?* I don't find any of this reassuring! Biotech industries are just as unregulated now as they were in the 1990s. So until I find out who's steering this ship, I'm buying only milk and soy that does *not* contain these unregulated genetically engineered proteins, which everybody says it is somebody else's job to regulate. And until our government and these corporations decide whose job it is to protect our health, I'll stick with milk labeled "organic" or "rBGH-free"—and you may want to do the same since, by law, these types of milk are not allowed to contain rBGH.

Monsanto and the Revolving Door

Actually, I thank my lucky stars that I *can* buy milk that's labeled "rBGH-free," because for more than a decade, Monsanto has been doing everything in its power to prevent companies from using that label. It was when I learned about *this* part of the story that I really started to lose sleep.

Let's go back to 1994, the year after rBGH was approved. Now it was time for Michael R. Taylor, FDA deputy commissioner for policy, to announce the FDA's labeling guidelines for this genetically altered milk protein.

Perhaps you think, as I did when I first read about this, that the FDA would be mainly concerned to label products that contained rBGH. Maybe they'd slap a label on rBGH milk saying, "Warning: could cause breast cancer," or "Made with genetically altered material," or even just "Contains added growth hormone" and let consumers figure it out for themselves. Or perhaps, worst-case scenario, the FDA would decide that products made with rBGH didn't have to be labeled at all.

But actually, the FDA went quite a bit further. Indeed, rBGH was *not* going to be labeled in milk. But in addition, the FDA basically restricted dairies that *didn't* use rBGH from pointing out that their milk was different from the genetically altered kind.

That's right. You didn't misread it. If a dairy wanted to highlight the fact that its milk had *not* been made with rBGH (you know, for those of us who might have an interest in avoiding this potentially carcinogenic hormone), the FDA recommended it to also state on the label that there was no difference between the genetically altered hormone that Monsanto had developed and the regular old bovine growth hormone that already occurred in nature.

Why did the FDA make such an extraordinary ruling? Because it didn't want rBGH milk to be "stigmatized" in the marketplace.

Are you as surprised as I was? Why in the world did the FDA seem so eager to protect Monsanto's interests?

Well, remember FDA deputy commissioner for policy Michael Taylor, who announced this policy? Guess where he had worked just before joining the FDA?

Not at a scientific institution. Not at another regulatory agency. Not at a highly respected university. At a law firm—Monsanto's law firm. Taylor had been a partner at King & Spaulding, the Washington, D.C., law firm that had represented Monsanto *while* the company was seeking FDA approval of rBGH. In fact, before leaving Monsanto's law firm and joining the FDA, Taylor had actually prepared a memo helping Monsanto figure out whether it could sue states or private businesses that wanted to label rBGH-free milk.

It gets worse. According to investigative researcher Jeffrey M. Smith, author of the internationally recognized book *Seeds of Deception,* the FDA actually created a new position for Taylor when it hired him in 1991. And after Taylor finished overseeing the regulatory approval of rBGH at the FDA, guess which company hired him on as vice president for public policy? Monsanto. Talk about a revolving door!

If Taylor were the only link between Monsanto and the FDA, that would be bad enough. But the revolving door kept spinning and the list goes on. Margaret Miller, for example, was a Monsanto researcher who prepared a report for the FDA asking the agency to find that rBGH was safe. Upon finishing her report at Monsanto, Miller left it to her colleagues to submit it to the FDA, while she went to work *for the FDA* as deputy director of the Office of New Animal Drugs, drugs like Posilac's rBGH. While at the FDA, Miller wrote papers on rBGH issues, some of which reached the desk of FDA commissioner David Kessler, to his later consternation when he learned of Miller's prior Monsanto connection.

Miller probably felt right at home at the FDA, because assisting her there was another former Monsanto-funded researcher, Susan Sechen. And Miller went right on taking Monsanto-friendly actions. For example, she also approved the hundredfold increase in the amount of antibiotics that farmers were allowed to give to cows. Remember, Posilac increases cows' risk of mastitis and other infections, so they need to be medicated far more often. Remember, too, that our kids' excessive exposure to antibiotics may be a significant factor in the allergy epidemic.

It's not as though the Monsanto-FDA connection went unnoticed. The General Accounting Office (GAO)—the congressional agency that addresses accountability of government agencies in budgetary matters—conducted an investigation of these ties in 1994. According to the GAO, though, the involvement of FDA officials in matters concerning their former employer did not constitute a conflict of interest. With all due respect to the GAO, I have to disagree.

Monsanto's efforts to protect the sale of rBGH milk didn't stop with the FDA. The giant corporation also made use of the electoral process and the court system. As I learned more about the influence that this corporation had over our government, I felt as though the world in which I was raised was now crumbling around me. Between that disillusionment and the research that I continued to unearth, I had given up on sleep almost entirely.

Punishing the Dairies

When Monsanto first introduced rBGH back in the 1990s, most Americans had never even heard of genetic engineering. As I said in chapter 3, I first learned of it on an August 2006 *Good Morning, America* segment with Diane Sawyer—and even at that late date, the respected and well-informed journalist seemed as shocked as I was.

But thanks largely to the Internet, knowledge had slowly started to spread. And so in 2002, a coalition of health-conscious organizations in Oregon tried to pass Measure 27, an initiative that would require all genetically engineered foods to be clearly labeled.

The corporations fought back. According to a Web site set up for the labeling campaign, www.voteyeson27.com, several companies, including Monsanto, kicked in some $6 million to ensure that the measure would be defeated, which it was.

The citizens were only asking for their right to know what was in their food. Apparently, Monsanto didn't think that *was* their right.

But Monsanto didn't stop there. In 2003, they went after Oakhurst, a small dairy in Maine. For the previous three years, Oakhurst had labeled its rBGH-free milk saying, "Our Farmers' Pledge: No Artificial Growth Hormones." Monsanto sued the company, which eventually had to add a second label, saying that "no significant difference has been shown between milk derived from (hormone)-treated and non-(hormone)-treated cows."

No significant difference? According to whom? The FDA, whose job it *wasn't* to test the safety of products sold by Monsanto? Or the Monsanto Corporation, whose job it *wasn't* to test the safety of products reviewed by the FDA?

Meanwhile, Monsanto had been requesting the FDA and the Federal Trade Commission (FTC) to go after dairies as well, punishing them for putting the "rBGH-free" label on their milk. The company was also working on the state level to oppose milk labeling. In fall 2007, they found an ally in Pennsylvania Secretary of Agriculture Dennis Wolff, who tried to prohibit the labeling of rBGH-free milk on the grounds that consumers were confused, even though a March 9, 2008, report in the *New York Times* said that Wolff's office "had no consumer research to back up his claim."

Ultimately, both consumer groups and Pennsylvania governor Ed Rendell opposed his efforts, and Wolff eventually had to back down. The state went on to "tighten . . . up the language on milk labels," according to the *Times* report.

Other states have considered tightening up their labeling language as well, including Indiana, Kansas, Missouri, New Jersey, Ohio, Utah, and Vermont. *Consumer Reports* published a survey in summer 2007 showing that some 88 percent of consumers want to allow dairies to label their rBGH-free milk. I guess Secretary Wolff missed that study.

But, as any corporation would, Monsanto apparently feared the loss of revenue that this rBGH backlash might create. So in fall 2007, it launched a new group to oppose the rBGH-free labeling effort called American Farmers for the Advancement and Conservation of Technology (AFACT).

When I read about AFACT, I thought perhaps they represented a genuine sector of the farm community. Then I learned that AFACT's members had, in fact, been organized by a public relations firm, Osborn & Barr Communications, which had been founded in 1988—with Monsanto as its sole client. The PR company now has other clients, including such agribusiness interests as John Deere, the United Soybean Board, and the Cattlemen's Beef Board/National Cattlemen's Beef Association. But Monsanto remains a key player, not least because company founder Steve Barr is a former Monsanto marketing executive, while founder Joe Osborn worked for the New York ad agency that handled Monsanto's accounts. Monsanto also contributes money to AFACT directly—or at least, it has while owning Posilac (the company's policy may change when it's no longer in the milk business).

By the way, AFACT isn't the only "mislabeled" consumer group out there. A group called the Center for Consumer Freedom frequently attacks the organic movement and groups who speak out against genetic engineering. It's funded by such well-known consumer advocates as Coca-Cola, Cargill (a major grain company), Tyson Foods, and—you guessed it—Monsanto. The group was founded by Berman & Co., a Washington, D.C.–based public affairs firm that also represents the tobacco industry, hotels, beer distributors, taverns, and restaurant chains.

Owner Rick Berman was the subject of a 2007 CBS News/60 *Minutes* report revealing that Berman's nickname in the industry is actually—I'm not making this up—"Dr. Evil." According to CBS, Berman's motto is "shoot the messenger": "getting people to understand that this messenger is not as credible as their name would suggest." In other words, if someone says that tobacco, beer, or, perhaps GM foods are bad for you, Berman's strategy is to attack that person's credibility, under the banner of consumer freedom.

So the next time you read about a group with a noble-sounding name attacking someone who's criticizing the food industry? Consider whether Dr. Evil may be lurking in the shadows pointing his high-powered sniper rifle right at the messenger.

The Milk Situation

So where do things stand, milkwise, as of this writing? Unfortunately, rBGH is still prevalent in much of our nation's milk supply. According to a March 25, 2008, article in the *Washington Independent,* "Most of the nation's leading dairy processors use milk from cows treated with the bovine growth hormone in at least some products," including Land O'Lakes, Good Humor, Breyers, Dreyer's, Dannon, Yoplait, and Sargento.

But I can also report—finally!—quite a bit of good news. It seems that consumers have found new ways to make their concerns heard, and at least some corporations are responding.

Of the 100 top U.S. dairy processors, 36 have declared themselves either partially or completely rBGH-free, including Kroger, Safeway Dairy Group, Anderson Erickson, and Publix Super Markets. Even Wal-Mart has announced that its private label, Great Value, milk will no longer come from Posilac-treated cows. And for over a decade, Ben & Jerry's ice cream containers have informed shoppers that the sweet treat is rBGH-free. And now Yoplait will be doing the same.

There's some more good news on the corporate front, as some food-processing companies are also breaking away from the use of rBGH-laden products. Dean Foods and Kraft, for example, offer some rBGH-free products, and Kraft is also planning to offer an entire rBGH-free product line. Retailers also are getting in on the trend: Starbucks went rBGH-free as of the end of 2007, as did Chipotle Restaurants.

As I learned about these corporations voluntarily removing this altered protein from their milk and dairy products, despite the FDA and Monsanto telling them that it wasn't necessary, I was inspired that perhaps all hope wasn't lost in the system that I had always supported. Unfortunately, there was another whole Monsanto manipulation that I had yet to learn about—one that shook my faith all over again.

Corn Bullies and the Monsanto Mafia

Monsanto doesn't just make rBGH. As I explained in chapter 3, it also manufactures Roundup, a top-selling herbicide used to spray a wide variety of crops, including corn, cotton, canola, alfalfa, sugar beets, and soybeans. You might have it in your garage, as it's sold to homeowners as well as farmers: it's one of the top-selling weed killers in the country.

Roundup wasn't the first weed killer that Monsanto made. In the 1960s, the company manufactured Agent Orange, used by the U.S. military to strip away the jungles of Vietnam. The company also made 2,4,5-T, another powerful herbicide.

But that was decades ago. Monsanto then expanded its product lines into agriculture and the growing fields of biotechnology and genetic engineering. In 1982, the company's scientists became some of the first to genetically modify a plant cell. The company was soon developing genetically modified crops—soybeans, corn, cotton, and canola, among others—that came onto the market during the 1990s. Robert Shapiro, president of the company during that extensive R&D process, called genetically modified (GM) seeds "the single most successful introduction of technology in the history of agriculture, including the plow."

At first, the two products—herbicide and genetically altered seeds—seemed to come from two different eras in the company's history. But slowly I realized that Monsanto had actually created a new kind of synergy: the genetically modified crops had actually been engineered to tolerate a super-sized portion of the company's own weed killer.

In a way, it sounded like a win-win. The new GM crops were doubly profitable for Monsanto, who could now sell more of its Roundup herbicide. And certainly, many in the farm community welcomed Monsanto's GM products, as this new technology claimed to promise increased profits through higher-yielding crops.

So in the United States, GM products spread rapidly through the fields, grocery stores, and food-processing companies, so that now, every time you or your family eats processed or packaged food, there's a good chance you're taking a bite of a genetically modified ingredient. Not a particularly appetizing thought once you know it, which may be why government agencies around the world were hesitant to embrace this technology and why Monsanto is so adamant about not having these ingredients labeled.

But it's not only consumers who suffer from Monsanto's high-handed ways. American farmers, too, pay a high price to the company. For millennia, farmers had saved the seeds from each year's crop to use for the next year. Now, with the introduction of genetically engineered seeds—patented technology belonging to Monsanto—the company had written new rules. If you want in on the GM "bonanza," the promises of bigger crops that the weeds or bugs can't get to, you can't save or store your own seed. Instead, you must buy new seeds from Monsanto every year.

What if you're a farmer who prefers *not* to try out the genetically engineered seeds? You, too, might end up with some Monsanto-inspired genetically altered crops on your land if the wind blows over some seed from your neighbor's crops or it is carried onto your land by birds. And what will happen if Monsanto investigators discover that you are in effect using Monsanto seeds without having actually paid for them?

Well, according to hundreds of farmers across the United States and Canada, what happens is that Monsanto comes after you with a court order, accuses you of stealing its property, and demands that you pay for the seeds that you "stole."

That's right. Even though you didn't take the seeds, didn't try to grow the seeds, maybe even didn't *want* the seeds, if they've made their way onto your property via wind, rain, the birds, or the bees, Monsanto says that your possession of those seeds has put you in violation of the law. No matter how those seeds got onto your land, Monsanto thinks you have to pay for them—and it's willing to take you to court to make its point.

When I've told friends about this corporate practice, they've found it hard to believe. "How does Monsanto even *know* that some seeds got onto your land?" one friend asked. "They would have to send investigators out to look for them."

I told her that's exactly what the company did. Hard as it is to believe, this $72 billion corporation actually hires investigators to travel through farm country and seek out "renegade crops" that might have sprung from Monsanto seeds. (I guess, with their corporate earnings, they can afford to.) Then the company has the crops analyzed and goes after the farmers who grow them. (I guess they can afford the court costs, too—though the farmers aren't always so lucky.)

I found it fascinating that the corporation would spend so much time and energy tracking down the effects of how the wind blows or how the birds and the bees fly, especially given that they had so quickly passed the buck on the safety issue to the FDA with the "Who's on First?" routine.

These actions have been documented in Deborah Koons Garcia's film, *The Future of Food,* as well as in a May 2008 *Vanity Fair* article, "Harvest of Fear," by Donald Barlett and James Steele. They wrote:

> As interviews and reams of court documents reveal, Monsanto re-
> lies on a shadowy army of private investigators and agents in the

American heartland to strike fear into farm country. They fan out into fields and farm towns, where they secretly videotape and photograph farmers, store owners, and co-ops; infiltrate community meetings; and gather information from informants about farming activities. Farmers say that some Monsanto agents pretend to be surveyors. Others confront farmers on their land and try to pressure them to sign papers giving Monsanto access to their private records. Farmers call them the "seed police" and use words such as "Gestapo" and "Mafia" to describe their tactics.

Monsanto refused to comment to *Vanity Fair* about its allegations, though it did say that the company had a stake in protecting its investment. They were starting to sound like the bully in my kids' lunchroom!

But I had more questions. How had the company been able to patent seeds? I was hardly an expert on patent law, but I'd always understood that patents were for inanimate objects. I hadn't realized you could patent a living thing or a potentially living thing, such as a seed or a plant. Given how many different ways plants could turn out, it seemed bizarre to think of patenting them.

I eventually learned that for most of its history, the U.S. Patent and Trademark Office had indeed refused to patent seeds. But in 1980, the U.S. Supreme Court ruled five to four that "a live human-made microorganism"—in this case, a bacterium invented by General Electric to clean up oil spills—could indeed be patented.

Monsanto made the most of this ruling, racking up 674 biotech patents—more than any other company. And so, when farmers buy Roundup Ready seeds, they are required to honor the patent by signing an agreement promising to neither save nor sell the seed. Unlike any tradition ever known in farm communities, farmers are required to buy new seed each year, rather than building up their own stock of seed from previous harvests. Talk about a recurring revenue stream for Monsanto!

This requirement has created a certain amount of confusion. Farmers may not understand that they're not allowed to save the seed, since that's what farmers have done pretty much since there *was* agriculture. Or they may balk at throwing perfectly good seed away. As we've seen, they might also end up with Monsanto seeds (and crops) on their land by accident. However it happens, they can count on one thing: Monsanto will come after them.

I (Reluctantly) Question Authority, Part 2

At this point, I guess, I'm glad to know what I've learned. On some level, it's always better to know the truth than to hide from it. But while I was going through this process, I was terrified. I just didn't know how to reconcile these horrifying new truths with the vision I'd always had of what it meant to be an American. I didn't know how to reconcile them with the idea I'd always had of corporations and our economic system. I would have given anything *not* to have to know all this, to go back to the same idealistic and maybe somewhat innocent person I'd been before.

This process led me to some dark days. They were all the darker for the gap they created between me and the family I came from. When I first began to find out about the corporate role in this story—the way Kraft had funded FAAN's Web site, the way the Peanut Foundation and Monsanto had funded the allergy doctors' research—I was knocked for a loop. I somehow felt responsible for sharing what I'd learned, but I didn't quite know how. So I turned, as I'd often done in times of uncertainty, to my dad.

My father is a strong, upright man who believes deeply in his country. He and my mom both served in Vietnam, but he'd always been the one to set the rules in our family—you might even say he's the one who lays down the law. My mother is the one who makes those rules work, trying to help us kids see how important it is to do what Dad thinks is right.

In the summer of 2006, my parents came out to see Jeff and me and the kids. One afternoon, I finally had the chance to tell Mom and Dad about the corporate connections I was uncovering.

"What am I supposed to do with this information?" I said when I had finished.

I wasn't really asking, though I guess deep down I maybe hoped that Dad would somehow have a magical answer that would make everything all better. But I wasn't at all prepared for what he did say, which was, "Nothing."

I looked at my father and thought, *Oh, Dad, that can't be your answer. How could I live with myself? I can't turn my back on my children like that.*

I looked at my father's set face, lined with years of concern, and realized that although his answer might have been born out of a desire to protect his daughter, he really *didn't* understand. To him, loyalty toward his country and our economic system meant that you didn't ask the kinds of questions that I wanted to ask—that I now felt I *had* to ask.

That afternoon I felt as though I had to make a choice between my parents' approval—Mom usually went along with Dad on these matters—and my devotion to my own kids. And my choice became immediately clear. I *had* to keep learning about the allergy epidemic and our government's role in it; I *had* to keep asking these questions about politics and the economy; and I *had* to share with other parents what I'd learned.

Given all that I had learned about the potential health risks in our food, how could I not fight for a mother's right to choose what to feed her family? If I walked away from that responsibility, how would I be able to look myself in the mirror ten years down the road? I was going to have to step out from underneath those roles, away from Dad's sternly protective arm.

So I let go of my parents' approval. I turned to my husband, and our four children. And I went forward.

5

CORN
CONTROVERSIES

The fall of 2006 was probably the hardest time in my life. I was saddened by the emotional separation from my mom and dad, which had somehow extended to my siblings as well. I was flooded with concern for the potentially lethal characteristics of the food that I had been feeding my family—food I had *thought* was safe.

I was falling deeper and deeper into despair, which I only realized through the change in my husband's attitude. Jeff had always been my pillar of strength, my cheerleader, my rock. Much of what I had learned was as upsetting to him as it was to me—he, too, had always believed in the integrity of our system—but he was always willing to listen, to keep an open mind, and to encourage me to keep moving forward.

But as the fall got colder and my mood got darker, Jeff became concerned. And one night, after putting the children to bed, I was overcome by a sense of incredible sadness for having inadvertently exposed my children to such a flood of chemicals. As I thought of the long-lasting damage that I might have caused them, I felt lost in a swamp of guilt. I was responsible, wasn't I? Even though I hadn't known any better, I had failed my children.

Jeff saw the huge burden of self-blame that I was taking on, and he tried to talk to me about it. When I finally saw how worried he was, I knew something had to change.

The next morning, I sat down at the breakfast table with my four children.

"You know how Mommy has been really busy with her computer lately?"

They all nodded.

"Well, Mommy is learning a lot of new things about chemicals in the food that we eat, and it makes me worried."

Five-year-old Colin quietly gave me a hug. John buzzed around the table, and six-year-old Lexy asked, "Is it about Tory's allergies?"

"Well, sort of. But it's not only Tory," I said. "There are chemicals in our food that might be bad for all of us. Now that I know this, I have to do something about it to protect all of you. And I have to help other people learn, so that their kids are safe, too."

This was the point when Colin absolutely floored me. He asked, "How many people are on your team?"

I almost had to laugh. "Not too many right now, Colin. But luckily I've got you, Lexy, John, Tory, and Daddy—that's my team."

Colin shook his head and looked me straight in the eye. "Mommy," he said, "you need a bigger team."

It was one of those moments when you realize that even a five-year-old can sometimes see things that you've missed. I *had* become far too isolated. I was learning some pretty uncomfortable things about FAAN, the medical establishment, and our government, things I really hadn't wanted to know. Now I saw that a lot of other people didn't want to know them either. People in the allergy community didn't want to know that the doctors on FAAN's medical board were also developing patents for Monsanto. Most of my friends didn't want to learn that their favorite comfort foods might actually be bad for their health, especially if they were used to thinking of them as health foods! And my parents and siblings didn't want to hear my concerns about the political and economic system in which they had always believed.

But surely there were other people out there, people who were already aware of the scope of the problem. Why couldn't I reach out to them?

I found the thought of writing to strangers both encouraging and daunting. I thought, Here I am, this mother of four in suburban Colorado, carpooling my kids to birthday parties and running to the grocery store. How can *I* get the word out about these financial relationships between our government and those giant corporations?

But I knew someone out there *would* understand. I just had to figure out who.

Then one day I saw a report on genetically modified foods that mentioned Nell Newman, the daughter of actor Paul Newman and the founder of Newman's Own Organics. I realized I had actually seen her face hundreds of times—it was her picture I saw on her brand's packaging.

Not only did I recognize Nell's name and face, but the Newman's Own business model—a for-profit business that gave all its proceeds to charity—had been so inspiring to me when I was starting my own business. Suddenly, I had one of those moments when the clouds part and you just *know* what your next step should be. Amateur as it might seem, I had to try to contact Nell through her company's Web site.

Wanting to appear as credible as possible—after all, I'd been in the business world and I knew you didn't approach someone out of the blue this way—I spent the next two days crafting that e-mail. I suspected that my chance of a reply was one in a million, but I had to start somewhere.

To my amazement, I got a personal response within less than a week from Nell Newman's own PR person, who told me she would make sure Nell heard about my work. Believe it or not, I found even this response incredibly empowering, because I suddenly realized that people might actually listen. Maybe I *could* convey this whole messy story in a way that people actually got. For the first time in a long time, I thought, *Maybe I can do this.*

When he got home that night, Jeff noticed right away that I had the stereo on. When I'd felt burdened by the depressing truths I was discovering, I couldn't bear to listen to music. Now, finally, I had reclaimed this source of comfort and joy, and for the first time in months, you could hear music in our house.

Even before I showed Jeff the e-mail from the Newman's Own team, he had begun to smile. And when I told him how relieved I felt that I might finally be able to *do* something about all the painful discoveries I had made, he nodded.

"I always knew you could," he said. Did I love this man or what?

The Allergy Detective Hunts Down the Corn Allergy

Besides genetically altered soy and milk, I was now on the trail of another genetically modified product—corn. I discovered that about 80 percent of the corn grown in the United States is genetically modified. Since corn is the largest U.S. crop, that's a lot of altered genes!

It's also a lot of corn. Corn growers are always on the lookout for new places to sell their product, and corn is currently used in a wide variety of food products—cereals, peanut butter, and snack foods—as well as in many nonfood products, including vitamins, aspirin, toothpaste, hairspray, deodorants, baby powder, cosmetics, and the ethylene often used to ripen fruits and vegetables. And, of course, ethanol.

As I had read in Michael Pollan's book *The Omnivore's Dilemma,* corn is also used to fatten up cattle. As a matter of fact, most of the corn and soy grown in the United States goes for livestock feed, but we humans end up consuming quite a bit of it, partly because corn lurks in places you'd never expect: lecithin, grain alcohol, vinegar, and ascorbic acid. It's even in the glue we lick on stickers and envelopes and the powder used to line latex gloves. Produce is often coated with a corn-based wax before shipping, and processed foods are generally preserved with such food additives as xantham gum, citric acid, maltodextrin, and dextrose (a.k.a. modified food starch), which can all be made from corn. If you wanted to avoid ingesting any form of corn, you'd have your work cut out for you.

Unfortunately, if you're one of those folks who suffer from corn allergy, that's exactly what you'd have to do. Even though some experts—and the folks at FAAN—don't even consider corn an allergen, the prestigious allergy researcher Dr. Samuel Lehrer has concluded that corn allergy does exist, although it is rare.

Dr. Lehrer, an associate professor at Tulane University Medical School, has conducted the only double-blind placebo-controlled corn allergy study, so it seems to me that he's the most informed expert out there on the topic. His work is further supported by some European studies, which point out that corn allergies may be more common in Africa and Central and South America, where corn plays a bigger part in the diet.

I had to wonder why the Europeans were doing a better job of researching this topic than we were in the United States. Meanwhile, Dr. Lehrer has been quoted as saying that he hopes FAAN will one day catch up with him and acknowledge the potential allergenicity of corn. Even more important is that the FDA should catch up, so that they can make sure that the labeling requirements in place for other allergens apply to corn as well.

Even though, according to the handful of small studies that have been conducted, only a small fraction of the population suffers from corn allergies, I didn't have to wonder why corn should concern *me*. I had just learned that Colin was allergic to it after he'd had a reaction at school. I had seen him suffer with immediate symptoms like rashes and a puffy face, and I had watched him come unglued the day after an attack, with inexplicable rages and inconsolable crying jags. He also suffered from headaches and stomachaches, which I knew made any emotional effects even worse. So I had to wonder whether, like allergies in general, the corn allergy was simply underdiagnosed.

Discovering the corn allergy was bad enough. When I first began to read about genetically modified corn, I felt like someone watching a horror movie: I was fascinated—and nauseated. Bad enough that soy had been genetically engineered to withstand herbicides. Corn had actually been genetically modified to contain its own insecticide in every cell and to release this insecticide as it grows! No wonder Coliin was allergic!

That's right. Genetically modified corn—technically known as Bt corn—has been scientifically altered to include the genetic code of an insecticide called Bt protein, a toxin that kills the corn rootworms that try to eat it. According to the College of Agriculture at the University of Kentucky, "Bt has been available as a commercial microbial insecticide since the 1960s and is sold under many trade names. These products have an excellent safety record and can be used on many crops until the day of harvest."

So this insecticidal toxin is safe to use on crops. But what about when the genetic material from these insecticides have been engineered *into* crops? If the scientists at the University of Kentucky tell me that I can consume a certain amount of poison without it hurting me, I suppose I can believe them—though I still wonder whether anyone has figured out the difference between cattle consuming the toxin in their feed and us humans (and our kids) consuming the toxins in the hundreds of places that corn is now used. But over and above my concerns about ingesting insecticide is another issue: the safety of the genetic engineering process itself.

To really understand what's going on with Bt corn, you need to know just what's going on inside those modified genes, as well as all the many, many things that can go wrong while the scientists tinker. So here's a short course in the how-tos of genetic engineering. You don't need to remember the details, but you do need to grasp the overview, because this is the operation that's being performed on a huge proportion of the food that you and your kids are eating. I promise to make the science a whole lot more fun than it was in high school—and this time, it's not an A on your term paper but your family's health that is at stake.

A Complicated Game of Telephone

The basic building block that scientists rely on for genetic engineering is—surprise, surprise—the *gene*. Think of the gene as a little piece of information, something that holds a *trait* that helps define an animal or a plant: the brown eyes you inherited from your father, for example, or the sweet-tasting sucrose inside a kernel of corn.

Genes are carried on long strands of DNA, which is short for *deoxyribonucleic acid.* You'll never have to remember that term again, so don't worry about it. What you should remember, though, is that along the long strand of DNA is a series of chemical compounds arranged into a complex pattern. The compounds are called *nucleotides.* Picture the nucleotides, arranged in their intricate genetic code. When you do, you'll begin to understand why genetic engineering is such a chancy proposition.

There are four types of nucleotides: adenine (A), thymine (T), cytosine (C), and guanine (G). Like long-lost lovers, the A and T always pair up, as do the C and G. You don't have to remember any of these details, but picture, for a second, a long strand of nucleotide pairs lined up along the DNA strand, maybe AT AT AT CG, or perhaps CG AT CG AT AT CG.

Now here's what you *do* need to remember: *Those patterns are the way your genes encode information.* Just as a computer reads long strands of ones and zeros, or as Morse code converts letters into dots and dashes, or as Braille spells out words with little dots, so does your pattern of ATs and CGs tell your DNA about all the complex traits you were born with. Remember how simple the little building blocks are—AT and CG are all we have to work with. Remember, too, how many complex and enormous patterns those simple little pairs can make.

So what do you think might happen to genetic information if a pattern gets disrupted or scrambled in ways we can't predict or detect? If we have a long sequence of ATs, for example, and someone thrusts a bunch of CGs right into the middle of them, what might the outcome be?

If you answered, *How should I know?,* well, give yourself an A-plus, because that's pretty much what a top genetic scientist would also have to answer. *We don't know what happens when we disrupt the genetic code.* We just don't know. When we insert foreign genetic material into a host gene, we might know what happens some of the time, or even most of the time. But nobody yet knows what happens *all* of the time. There are just too many variables.

Let's go back to that long strand of DNA. In order to pass the genetic code on to its descendants, it goes through a complex, three-stage process. Think of it as an extremely complicated game of telephone, in which an incredibly detailed and important message has to get whispered from one person to the next.

1. *Transcription:* The DNA passes a message to "messenger RNA."
2. *Translation:* The messenger RNA passes the information to a protein.
3. *Expression:* The protein then expresses the trait encoded in the DNA.

Why is *this* important? *Because again, something can go wrong every step of the way.* You've got the transcription process. You've got the translation process. And you've got the protein prepared to express—or perhaps, to suppress—all that genetic information. When you think about this remarkably complex and delicate series of events, it's kind of amazing that it doesn't go wrong more often, even when we humans are *not* consciously trying to influence it!

Of course, sometimes the process *does* go wrong. Genes *mutate,* or change in unexpected ways. Messages get mixed up. Genetic material does unpredictable things, creating deformities, rare diseases, or creatures that can't survive. Most of the time, though, genes pass on useful information from one generation to the next, and the species soldiers on.

Here's another amazing thing about genes: they've got natural barriers against genetic material from other species. In nature, you can't mate a cat with a dog, for example. Even if you could artificially inseminate one animal with sperm from another, the genes wouldn't mesh. If you wanted to create a "dat" or a "cog," you would have to find an approach that somehow breaks through the barriers that nature has provided.

Likewise, you can't cross-pollinate, say, an oak with a violet. No matter how much violet pollen blows onto the oak, the two plants are simply not going to breed. If you wanted to make a purple oak or a ten-foot-high violet, you would have to find some new method to get the genes to mesh, because nature will fight you every step of the way.

Why is *that* important? Because that is one of the major differences between regular old conventional breeding—trying to breed a fatter cow, for example, or a sweeter ear of corn, or a hardier tomato—and genetic engineering. Almost every existing version of conventional breeding combines the genetic material from two organisms that are already pretty close, unable to breach these natural barriers. Only genetic engineering brings two wildly different creatures—a tomato and a scorpion, a corn plant and a bacterium—together.

True, conventional breeding does include a technique called "wide breeding," in which the two organisms are a bit further apart. But even in wide breeding, the life-forms are very much like each other. You couldn't combine a peach and a watermelon, let alone a peach and a scorpion.

Yet in one especially creepy-sounding version of genetic engineering, the DNA for scorpion toxin is inserted into tomato genes to help the tomatoes fight off bugs. That's on a whole other level from anything that could happen in nature. And again, nobody yet knows all the things that might go wrong at this level, because never, in the history of the planet, has it ever happened, at least, not until Monsanto created the first genetically engineered protein in 1982.

When I got to this point in my own effort to understand genetic engineering, I was wondering, *If nature is designed to prevent certain species from crossing, how in the world do they get the different genes to mix?* It's actually kind of fascinating, in a science-fiction kind of way. These days, there are two widely used methods: the virus and the gene gun.

Viruses and Gene Guns

Gene guns are pretty much what they sound like. Scientists use a gun-like instrument to shoot, say, microscopic pellets of gold into a gene. The gold particles are coated with DNA from the new trait, and when the process works, the DNA is incorporated into the host cell. The gold is basically needed only for the gun to have something "weighty" to shoot; the DNA is too light to travel by itself.

Another way to accomplish this process is by using some type of bacteria like a harmless salmonella strain or a virus, like *e. coli,* to penetrate the host cell. After all, that's what bacteria and viruses do: they sneak into places where they're not always wanted—as in the case of an infection—and set up housekeeping. If the salmonella or *e. coli* are carrying some foreign DNA—which is unlikely to happen in nature but which can happen in a laboratory—they can "infect" the host cell's genes with their new DNA.

So picture all these host cells—maybe from a soybean plant, maybe from an ear of corn—sitting in their petri dishes, shot up with gene guns or "infected" by bacteria or viruses. Because this process is so unnatural—because it goes against all the defenses that the cell has set up—it's not going to work very often. It might work only once every several thousand times, or maybe even one in a million times.

So what the scientists want to do next is to identify those few cells that were transformed and move on to the next stage, *regeneration*. This is the part where they actually create a new transgenic plant from a single transformed cell.

But wait, before we go on to that remarkable stage, how do we know which cells have been transformed and are therefore worth regenerating? No point in creating plants that are just like the ones we already have. We're only interested in regenerating the cells that have been transformed. So we need some way to identify those happy few on whom the experiment worked.

Scientists came up with a clever solution for that problem, known as a *marker gene,* which travels with the gene they really care about—the one that kills insects, for example. It's hard to know whether the insecticide gene has made it into the cell, but it should be easy to identify the marker gene. Nowadays, for example, the marker gene might make the cell glow a bright fluorescent green. If you see a green glowing cell, you know that both the marker gene and the insecticide gene have transferred their DNA into the cell.

Back in the 1990s, in the early days of genetic engineering, the marker gene was often a gene for resistance to antibiotics. Remember, antibiotics kill most bacteria—that's what they were designed to do. But if the bacterium used in the genetic engineering process is *resistant* to antibiotics, it will survive the medication. So genetic engineers put some "resistance gene" into each little genetic package (they actually call it a *cassette*). Then they sprayed all the cells with antibiotics. The antibiotics killed the cells that hadn't been transformed, and the engineers harvested the rest.

Of course, you can see the problem right away, can't you? Do we really want to be promoting the spread of bacteria that are resistant to antibiotics? What happens if those resistant bacteria get into our digestive systems, which might happen when we eat the genetically altered plant? And what if we then pick up an infection that our doctor wants to treat with antibiotics? There's at least some chance that we'll resist the antibiotic's effects.

I should assure you that the genetic engineers are careful to pick "resistance" genes linked to antibiotics that we humans don't really need. So everyone, even the most severe critics of genetic engineering, agrees that the risks are probably small.

Still, there is *some* risk. That's why the World Health Organization and other agencies have said that antibiotic-resistance markers should be phased out, and nowadays they're rarely used. Still, one major concern about genetic engineering is that there are still plenty of plants out there passing on antibiotic resistance down to their descendants—and maybe, also, to ours.

Meanwhile, back at the lab, there is yet another element that we need to include in our little genetic cassette. We've already got the transformed gene, known as the *transgene* for short, carrying the new trait we want to insert, such as the ability to kill some insects. And we've got the *marker gene,* which lets us know that the transformation process has worked. Now we need a *promoter,* something that will help the new genetic material express itself in the new plant that we're about to create.

To understand the promoter, picture your genes as elements in a recording studio. You've got this huge dimmer board that controls the volume of thousands of different elements—vocals, violins, drums, guitars. You can turn some elements up very loud, keep others at medium levels, and soften others so much that they basically aren't heard at all.

It's the same with genes. Every organism has way more genetic *potential* than it expresses. Some of its genes are turned up very loud and their expression pretty much dominates that organism's identity. Some of its genes are a bit quieter, or perhaps they vary from loud to soft to medium depending on the circumstances. And some are completely silent.

For example, expression of the gene for melanin (skin pigment) varies a great deal. In dark-skinned people, the melanin gene is always expressing itself, and the skin stays dark. In fair-skinned people, the melanin gene is pretty quiet—until, perhaps, the sun comes out. Then all those light people who are capable of tanning will turn up the volume on their melanin gene and watch their skin turn brown. When the sun retreats, the melanin gene gets quieter and the skin color lightens again.

So if you were creating a new transgene, one that was going to add a whole new quality to the host cell, would you want one with the volume turned up or down? Usually, you'd want that volume turned up, enough to drown out the music that the old gene usually plays—and for that, you need a *promoter.*

Think of the promoter as the dial on your stereo or the movable switch on a sound board. You use it to turn the volume up as high as it will go, so the newly inserted gene expresses itself as loudly as possible.

The promoter that's usually used for genetically engineered corn is a kind of bacteria called the *Agrobacterium tumefaciens*. This bacterium causes crown gall disease by creating galls—ugly tumor-like growths.

As you can see, the bacterium is useful for genetic engineering, because it causes cells to reproduce at a furious pace, thus creating the tumor-like growth, the gall. The crown gall virus turns up the volume on the insecticide that's been added to the corn, causing the corn to produce more insecticide cells, so that its new genetic potential to kill insects is fully expressed.

There's one more piece of the genetic cassette that you need to know about, and that's what scientists call the *termination sequence*. I think of it as the off switch, myself. It's the code that tells the gene to *stop* doing what it's doing.

Okay. Now you've heard how genetic engineering is *supposed* to work. It's a complex process, I know, so here's a quick and easy review:

1. A gene gun or bacterium *inserts* new genetic material into a bunch of host cells.

2. A tiny fraction of the host cells accepts the new material and incorporates it into their own genes.

3. If the process works, the gene is transformed. The original DNA *transcribes* its message into the RNA. The RNA *translates* the message into a protein. And presto! A new genetically engineered protein is born!

4. That protein *expresses* itself as a new trait—maybe resistance to insects or to herbicides.

5. The *promoter* turns up the volume on that expression.

6. The termination sequence *turns off* the instructions to express the trait. And the new plant lives happily ever after, reproducing the new trait for generations to come. That's what happens when the process goes right. But what happens when something goes wrong?

When Good Genes Go Bad

To understand how and why genetic engineering goes wrong, all you have to do is picture the incredibly complex process that's involved. Then remember this sentence: *Something can go wrong every step of the way.*

Part of the problem is that we don't know exactly *where* into the host gene we are inserting the new genetic material. So right off the bat, there are three ways things can go off course:

1. *The new material we are inserting may get scrambled, sending a different message than we intended.* We tell the new plant to become more resistant to insects, for example, and it just doesn't hear the message clearly.

This happens sometimes with GM crops: the actual plants don't always fulfill their promises. According to one study, the new insect-resistant Bt cotton failed to provide the promised insect control in up to 50 percent of the acreage. The Texas farmers who bought the seed actually sued its maker, Monsanto, and won, but the terms of their settlement mean they can't talk about what happened.

2. *The insertion process itself may change something in the host gene.* This scary possibility is called *insertional mutagenesis,* and it, too, has actually happened.

In 2003, eleven French patients were being treated with genetically engineered proteins that were inserted into their bone marrow cells with the worthy goal of treating their immune deficiency. But the insertion created a new problem: somehow, three of those eleven patients developed leukemia. In trying to cure one disease, the genetic engineers had apparently induced the patients to develop another.

In 2005, a researcher at the National Institutes of Health had a similar experience with a primate, who came down with leukemia five years after undergoing gene transfer. Another side effect of the process was that the animal developed resistance to certain forms of chemotherapy.

3. *While we are changing one trait, we may end up changing others that we don't intend to change.* The scientific term for that is *pleiotropy,* and it occurs because genes are so complex.

Genetic engineers used to think genes were simple, and that we could put them together and take them apart like Legos. In reality, genes are way more complicated. Instead of resembling Legos, which remain more or less discrete even when connected, they're more like members of a little ecosystem in which all the different parts interact. Introduce one new plant or animal or insect into that ecosystem, and suddenly everything goes haywire. This doesn't always happen with genetic engineering. But it certainly happens sometimes.

So far, I've told you what can go wrong with the *insertion* of the new genetic material, which is the first stage of the genetic engineering process. But as you recall, the process has two more stages: *transcription* and *translation.* A wide variety of things can go wrong with those stages, too.

Yet another place where things can go wrong is the *termination code.* If this code gets messed up—and with our clumsy insertion process, that's bound to happen sometimes—the plant might produce *too* much of something or start growing out of control. Or the termination code for some other process might get disrupted. Perhaps a plant is supposed to produce something only in certain quantities or at certain times of the year. With a faulty termination code, the plant might behave in unpredictable and problematic ways.

Remember the long strand of DNA, decked out in pairs of ATs and CGs? Think again of how complex the codes are—all the many different patterns that the AT/CG pairs can make. Now imagine shoving some new AT/CG patterns in the midst of it all, shot in by a gene gun or carried in by a bacterium. How many ways could the code get messed up? What might all the consequences be?

You don't need to remember the details of this already oversimplified explanation. But here are the points I *would* like you to take away:

1. Genes are incredibly complicated.
2. Genes interact with one another, and with their environment, in complex and unpredictable ways.
3. Genetic engineering may work most of the time—but no one can guarantee that it will work all of the time.
4. When it doesn't work, we don't yet know what will happen.

When I got to this point in my own reading, my head was spinning. I had to take a break from all that science and focus on something concrete. Luckily—or unluckily—I could read about a real-life example of genetic engineering gone wrong: the story of the StarLink scandal.

The StarLink Scandal

The StarLink scandal is a fascinating example of how genetic engineering and the allergy epidemic are potentially linked. StarLink was a genetically engineered form of corn that was created by the France-based Aventis company. The GM corn was never meant to feed humans—it had been created as animal feed—but by September 2000, it had somehow found its way into the human food supply and ended up in Taco Bell taco shells, which are distributed by Kraft Foods, Inc. StarLink corn flour was also detected in taco shells manufactured by Mission Foods of Irving, Texas, whose Taco Bell products are relabeled with store-brand packaging for Safeway, Food Lion, Shaw's, and several other grocery chains. According to the FDA's Center for Food Safety and Applied Nutrition, the allergenic corn might even have made its way into the beer supply!

As often happens with these things, no one knew there was a problem until a bunch of people started getting sick. It's difficult to determine how many people got sick and with what symptoms, because although the Centers for Disease Control and the FDA investigated StarLink, they never did a comprehensive study. Instead, they tested the blood of seventeen people who had reported a range of symptoms that resembled allergic reactions, from upset stomachs to anaphylactic shock. Since they didn't find any IgE antibodies to StarLink corn in their subjects' blood, they concluded that the corn had not provoked an immune-system reaction.

As you remember from chapter 1, IgE antibodies are the sign that you have an allergy: they're what your immune system makes to defend against proteins that it perceives as toxic invaders. The government agencies concluded that without the presence of IgE antibodies in the blood of those few people whom they tested, StarLink could not be a true allergen.

However, another government agency came up with a slightly different conclusion. On July 19, 2001, the Environmental Protection Agency's scientific advisory panel determined that although the previous investigation had shown that certain *individuals* were not allergic to StarLink, those findings didn't mean that *no one* could be allergic to StarLink. The EPA panel also criticized the other agencies for not having investigated the possibility that there were lots of people out there who *had* had allergic reactions to StarLink—but who hadn't reported them.

Meanwhile, StarLink corn was in trouble. Grain importers around the world were suddenly reluctant to accept American shipments, for fear of contamination. And indeed, when grain elevators and food companies tested their incoming shipments of corn, they found it difficult to be certain that no trace of potentially fatal StarLink was included. A Cornell-based group called the Public Issues Education Project concluded that "Although StarLink corn was less than 1% of the total 1999 and 2000 corn harvest, mixing of StarLink with other corn varieties at individual mills may have caused a disproportionately larger number of corn products to be contaminated."

The whole StarLink scandal raised lots of questions about genetically engineered foods. As we've seen, Dr. Hugh Sampson, one of the nation's leading allergists, was part of a panel convened by the EPA in late 2000 to investigate the safety of StarLink corn.

(By the way, if you're wondering why the EPA and not the FDA was regulating StarLink, it's because StarLink corn was considered an insecticide. After all, it had been genetically engineered to contain its own insecticidal toxins. Since the FDA regulates food while the EPA regulates insecticides, the matter was given to the EPA, which regulates all of the GM insecticidal corn that we eat for the same reason.)

Dr. Sampson, to his credit, spoke out loud and clear about the many unknowns inherent in the StarLink situation. "[N]obody can say for sure that a new protein won't be a problem," he said frankly.

As I had thought when I first stumbled on the GM-allergy link, there *was* at least a potential connection between the introduction of new proteins and the allergy epidemic. Although Dr. Sampson had dismissed this theory when I had asked my fellow allergy mom to present it to him two years ago, here were his own words from only nine years ago, warning of the same dangers I was concerned about. What had happened to this man?

Then I remembered that Dr. Sampson had gone on to develop a patent designed to increase the insecticidal activity in the genetically modified potato, for perhaps the largest biotech company on earth—Monsanto. *Oh,* I thought. *Maybe that's what happened.* I couldn't help but wonder how his role as coinventor of the 2005 patent had affected his ability to candidly address this issue, as he had in 2000. (For more on Dr. Sampson's involvement with Monsanto, see chapter 7.)

Meanwhile, a number of consumer groups were publishing criticisms of the EPA's StarLink investigation. Some groups came right out and said that the EPA's study was just one big whitewash. Here are a few of the main objections raised by such organizations as Friends of the Earth and Genetically Engineered Food Alert, a coalition of environmental groups.

1. *Not enough people were tested.* The seventeen people tested by the FDA tested negative for allergies. But many critics felt that the sample was too small, considering that millions of people had

been exposed to StarLink, and that hundreds of people had made corn-related allergy complaints after the StarLink scandal was reported. Experts recommended that the medical and allergy communities be monitored, so as to uncover any additional cases of exposure to StarLink. But the EPA chose not to do so.

2. *The wrong testing method was used.* The genetically engineered protein in StarLink corn is known as Cry9C, so this was the protein they needed to test for allergic reactions. As with most allergy tests, participants were injected with a small amount of the potential allergen. Then their blood was examined to see if it contained IgE antibodies to the protein.

But there's a wrinkle. Because the protein is genetically engineered—because it isn't found in nature—it can come in two forms: engineered into the food, so that it develops as the corn grows, and engineered in the lab, as a kind of copy of what you might find in nature. When the EPA conducted its test, it didn't use the form of Cry9C that actually appears in a kernel of GM corn. Instead, it used a laboratory version of Cry9C.

Critics pointed out that the two versions of Cry9C—grown in the corn and grown in the lab—are *not* identical. The laboratory version has far fewer sugar molecules. And often, the critics said, it's precisely those extra sugar molecules that can make a protein more allergenic.

Accordingly, the critics claimed that the test results were skewed. Instead of testing people with the most allergenic form of the protein—the one engineered into the food that they would actually have been exposed to—the EPA tested them with the one made in the laboratory, an apparently milder form that contained fewer sugar molecules. Could that have been the reason that none of the seventeen subjects reacted?

3. *Special risks to infants, children, and farmworkers were not considered.* Health hazards don't affect everybody equally. Some people—especially infants and children—are more at risk. As we

know, children are more allergic than adults, as they may outgrow some or all of their allergies by the time they've reached adulthood. So if the EPA really wanted to know whether StarLink provoked allergic reactions, shouldn't it have tested children?

Children's health was a special concern because hypoallergenic infant formulas—formulas made especially for kids with allergies—often contain corn. Mead Johnson's Enfamil Nutramigen, for example, was 54 percent cornstarch and corn syrup solids, according to the environmental group Friends of the Earth. Yet the government never tested any infant formulas to see if they contained the allergy-inducing proteins.

Another vulnerable group was the farmworkers who had grown StarLink corn. Remember, StarLink corn was Bt corn: it contained the Bt toxin, intended to kill insects. According to EPA tests in a completely separate study, farmworkers in fields sprayed with Bt toxins had immune-system reactions apparently caused by breathing in the toxin. Wouldn't farmworkers also be more likely to respond to a day spent in the fields with Bt corn? Shouldn't the EPA have investigated this possibility as part of their decision to regulate StarLink? But like infants and children, the farmworkers were ignored.

So although it started with a bang, the StarLink scandal ended with a fizzle, its potential significance buried—like the secrets of the Lost Ark—in a bureaucratic basement full of documents that only a few maverick researchers keep insisting on bringing to light. Luckily, we haven't had another such scandal since then, so you might be tempted to conclude that the system works. But based on what I've learned about genetic engineering, the FDA, the EPA, and the agribusiness and processed food companies who dominate the market, I keep on waiting for the other shoe to drop. Or when you consider the skyrocketing figures of the allergy epidemic and food recalls, maybe it already has.

Genes Gone Wild

Having learned some of the basics of genetic engineering and having seen how badly things went wrong in the StarLink scandal, I was now forced to confront what our government was and was not doing to protect our health and the health of our children. One of my first steps was reading a document written by Michael Hansen, PhD.

Dr. Hansen is a scientist with the Consumer Policy Institute of the Consumers Union, and he's spent a lot of time thinking about safety issues and genetic engineering. Back in 2003, he wrote a memo called "Reasons for Caution About Introducing Genetically Engineered Corn in Africa: Food Safety Issues." I guess having witnessed the StarLink fiasco firsthand, Dr. Hansen felt a responsibility to convey how things could go terribly wrong, especially to countries who didn't even have an Environmental Protection Agency.

I thought, when I read his document, that his reasons for urging caution certainly applied to our country as well. After all, genetic engineering was a whole new industry—and yet, we hadn't ever really taken the steps we needed to understand how it worked, let alone to regulate it.

So here's what Michael Hansen thinks is problematic about the way we regulate genetic engineering:

THE FDA DOESN'T REQUIRE SAFETY TESTING FOR GENETICALLY ENGINEERED PLANTS. To understand how this happened, think back to 1992, when President George H. W. Bush and Vice President Dan Quayle were working to deregulate as many sectors of the economy as they could to provide regulatory relief to industry. As part of that deregulation process, according to a January 25, 2001, article in the New York Times, "Mr. Quayle told a crowd of executives and reporters in the Indian Treaty Room of the Old Executive Office Building, 'We will ensure that biotech products will receive the same oversight as other products, instead of being hampered by unnecessary regulation.'" Despite growing concerns among scientists within the government agency, the FDA accepted Quayle's proposal rather than insisting on funding for the development of new testing methods.

At the time, some courageous FDA scientists spoke out in favor of regulating genetic engineering. "This is the industry's pet idea, that there are no unintended effects that will raise the F.D.A.'s level of concern," wrote Dr. Louis J. Pribyl, one of the government scientists charged with developing a policy for genetically engineered foods. "But time and time again, there is no data to back up their contention."

Likewise, three FDA toxicologists wrote, "The possibility of unexpected, accidental changes in genetically engineered plants justifies . . . study."

But the voices of protest were ignored. Deregulation was further advanced under the Clinton-Gore administration when they were elected later that year. Now the FDA's view is that since you don't need to safety-test the plants bred by conventional methods, you don't need to test the ones created through genetic engineering, either.

However, we've seen that genetic engineering is a far riskier business than conventional plant breeding. Do we really think it's okay to simply rely on corporate testimony, rather than specifically testing new GM plants? According to researchers at the University of Kentucky, Bt corn hybrids (the ones containing the genes for an insecticidal protein) differ from conventional plants in many ways. Yes, they contain the Bt protein, but genetic engineering has created other differences as well. Yet the FDA treats Bt corn and regular corn as though they were the same—and concludes that because regular corn doesn't need to be regulated, Bt corn doesn't either.

THE FDA ADMITS THAT ITS ORIGINAL POLICY WAS BASED ON A FALSE NOTION. The 1992 FDA policy, as we just saw, was based on the notion that genetic engineering really isn't that different from conventional breeding—that it produces plants that are "substantially equivalent" to conventional ones. Many scientists no longer think that way—and, as of 2001, neither does the FDA. In 2001, the FDA referred to possible "unintended changes" that could result from genetic engineering, implicitly acknowledging the many ways genetic engineering could go wrong. Yet it did not implement any new requirements that industries test for "unintended changes" before receiving FDA approval for their GM plants.

A MAJOR FOOD SAFETY CONCERN FOR GENETICALLY MODIFIED PLANTS IS ALLERGENICITY. As you recall from our discussions in chapters 2, 3, and 4, genetic engineering consists of the insertion of foreign proteins into places where they would not naturally occur. This insertion process literally creates new proteins. Since this process was introduced into our food supply in 1994, scientists have been concerned that these new proteins might be allergenic. Remember all those discussions sponsored by the FDA, the StarLink scandal, and the concerns expressed by former FAAN chair Dr. Fred McDaniel Atkins? This is what all those scientists were worried about—and their concerns were shared by the U.N.'s Food and Agriculture Organization, as well as its World Health Organization, which developed a protocol for figuring out whether new genetically altered foods might cause allergies. But *none* of the genetically altered crops on the U.S. market—including Bt corn—have been tested according to that protocol. True, any effective testing will be unwieldy and expensive. Since genetically modified foods are so unpredictable, it's difficult even to know what to test for. This is exactly why Europe follows the precautionary principle: as long as you don't know how it's going to affect us, don't put it in our food.

COUNTRIES AROUND THE WORLD HAVE AGREED ON WHAT COUNTS AS A PROPER "SAFETY ASSESSMENT" OF GENETICALLY MODIFIED FOODS—BUT NO GENETICALLY ALTERED U.S. CROP HAS ACTUALLY BEEN STUDIED THAT WAY. If we're not testing genetically altered corn, soy, and other crops, how do we know they're safe? And until we do figure out which ones are safe, shouldn't we follow the precautionary principle upheld in Europe, Australia, Russia, and Japan, stating that if something hasn't been proven safe, you just can't use it?

THERE'S EVIDENCE THAT BT CORN DOES CONTAIN A GENETICALLY ENGINEERED ALLERGEN. As we saw with the StarLink scandal, Bt corn includes toxins known as Cry proteins. These same proteins are also found in Bt pesticide sprays. And as we saw a few pages ago, these Bt sprays have produced allergy-like symptoms among farmworkers.

THERE ARE TOXINS IN BT FOODS THAT RESEMBLE KNOWN HUMAN ALLERGENS. In 1998, FDA head of biotechnology studies Dr. Steve Gendel found that there's a close resemblance between some proteins found in Bt corn and Bt cotton, and an allergen found in egg yolk protein (vitellogenin). There's also a resemblance between a Bt potato protein and a major milk allergen (beta-lactoglobulin). So there *is* a chance that genetically altered foods can be allergenic—but the FDA doesn't require corporations to test for that possibility.

THE PROTEINS IN BT CORN AFFECT THE IMMUNE SYSTEM. A series of studies conducted in Mexico and Cuba suggests that one of the Bt corn's proteins created immune-system problems and allergy symptoms among mice. Again, the FDA doesn't require companies to test for these problems. Clearly, more testing needs to be done—but who's going to make sure that it is?

Dr. Hansen also shared with me a second paper, written by Joe Cummins, professor emeritus of genetics at the University of West London, Ontario, and an international expert in environmental concerns and genetic engineering. Like many concerned scientists, Professor Cummins was disturbed by the inadequate regulatory processes in North America, which he attributes to faulty assumptions on the part of the regulators. For example, he points out that the Bt toxin has been introduced into a number of different plants (as we've seen, into corn, cotton, sugar beets, and potatoes, among others). Regulators, he says, evaluate only the Bt toxin itself—not the form it takes within the plant.

"Regulators have simply assumed that the toxins produced using the altered synthetic genes are equivalent to the natural gene toxin," he writes.

In fact, the altered synthetic genes are *not* the same as the natural toxin. As we just saw, all sorts of things can change when new genetic material is inserted into that long, complicated DNA strand with all its AT and CG pairs. Regulators have to evaluate the gene in its new, synthetically altered form, not its old, natural form.

But this has not been done, because, says Professor Cummins, "the cost of isolating the toxins from the GM crops was considered prohibitive." Well, speaking as the mother of four children, I think that *not* testing those new genes may have a cost that is even more prohibitive. What do you think? And given that Monsanto is worth $72 billion as of the writing of this book, don't you think that they could use some of their record profits on additional R&D and develop some tests to ensure the safety of the brand-new proteins they have created? True, any effective testing will be unwieldy and expensive. Since genetically modified foods are so unpredictable, it's difficult even to know what to test for. So maybe we should follow Europe's lead and use the precautionary principle here in the United States: until you know how it's going to affect us, don't put it in our food.

Professor Cummins also discusses the environmental problems of genetic engineering. For example, he writes, "The soil around the GM crop may accumulate toxins, if these are released to the soil." In fact, Bt toxin has been found in the litter around Bt corn plants, and in one study, worms exposed to that toxic litter experienced a large weight loss.

Now I'll admit, when I first read about this, I thought, *Why in the world should I care about skinny worms?* Then I learned that we rely on worms to aerate the soil and allow plants to grow. I already knew that one of the unintended consequences of genetic engineering might be the rise in the allergy epidemic. What if another unintended consequence was that it weakened or eventually killed off creatures on whom we depend to protect our food out in the fields?

It isn't only worms who may be affected by genetic engineering. Beneficial predators—the insects that we count on to eat *other* insects—may also be destroyed by Bt crops, according to Professor Cummins, who adds that "their loss would be costly."

The green lacewing, for example, eats insect pests that feed on corn. But if the pests have eaten Bt toxins, what happens to the lacewings? Studies have shown that in the vicinity of GM crops, many lacewings died and others suffered from delayed development. It's not clear whether the lacewings were responding to the Bt toxin itself or to some by-product of the genetic engineering process—but it is clear that the Bt corn was killing them off.

Now, I'm no tree hugger, and I'm certainly not an insect lover. Houston is full of mosquitos, and I grew up religiously spraying myself with OFF. So I didn't immediately see why I should care about lacewings, either.

Then I realized that if the insects who eat *other* insects are destroyed, almost the only remaining way to kill insects will be through pesticides—chemical compounds that we will *have* to buy from Monsanto and other corporations. Do we really want a situation in which almost all the natural ways to prevent insects have been destroyed, so that we are virtually dependent on genetic engineering, chemicals, and insecticides?

I turned to one of our top agriculturalists, Dr. John P. Reganold, PhD, Regents Professor of Soil Science, Department of Crop and Soil Sciences, Washington State University. He worked for two years as a soil scientist with the U.S. Department of Agriculture's Natural Resource Conservation Service and for three years as an environmental engineer with Utah International, Inc., a mining company. Now he's one of the world's premier scientists in sustainable agricultural research, as evidenced by his publications in *Science, The Economist, Nature, Proceedings of the National Academy of Sciences (PNAS), Scientific American,* and other journals.

Through a friend's introduction, Dr. Reganold had quickly become a mentor in this brave new world, so I asked him if he knew of evidence of bees being harmed by genetically engineered crops. He immediately sent over an article on wild bees and canola crops (remember, canola is one of the largest genetically modified crops along with soy, corn, and cotton).

According to the article, prepared by biologists at Simon Fraser University in British Columbia, bee populations declined in the vicinity of genetically modified crops and flourished around traditional crops. Could this possibly help explain the noted decline of the bee population?

Finally, Professor Cummins points out that animals who consume Bt corn may be retaining both the toxin and the altered DNA in their digestive systems. There is some evidence that cows fed on genetically modified fodder have died, and that the Bt toxin and transgenic DNA may survive in the intestines of mice, causing intestinal and immune system changes.

Now, think about that for a minute. If cows fed on Bt corn are not fully digesting the toxins, does that mean *we* absorb the toxins when we eat the meat from those cows or drink their milk? Does it mean that *we* absorb the toxins if we eat the corn, as seems to have happened with StarLink (even though that corn was never intended for human consumption)? Does it mean that *we* absorb the toxins if they end up in the litter around the corn and then somehow migrate to a nearby field where food that we will consume is grown?

So many questions—and so few answers. So I'll repeat my most important questions: *Why aren't the studies being done? And, why aren't we at least living up to the standards set by Europe, Australia, Japan, and even Russia, and labeling or banning these products until they are further studied?*

Actually, there is one bright note on the horizon. Because of a firestorm of bad publicity about genetic modification, McDonald's, Burger King, and Pringles all decided not to use GM spuds in their French fries and chips. They made that decision all the way back in 2000—even as GM corn, soy, and other products continued to be ever more widely used. So our children's Happy Meals can make us at least a little bit happy, even while we have to ask, *Why aren't other U.S. corporations equally concerned about protecting our kids?*

Giant Steps

As I came to terms with what I'd been learning—about genetic engineering, about Monsanto, about our government, about our country—I also had to come to terms with my own relationship to the food industry. This wasn't some abstract political issue; this was the food I fed my kids and my husband, the food I ate myself. The idea that these corporations, these policies, these chemicals and altered genes had taken up residence under my roof and in our bodies was, at times, over-whelming. Not to mention that on top of all that, I had also learned about the money that the USDA was paying to farmers to give them fi-nancial incentives to grow these chemical-laden crops. If they could sub-sidize genetically engineered corn for the hamburger bun in a Happy Meal, why couldn't they subsidize unmodified corn for a better bun in a healthy meal?

One day, I felt I'd simply had enough. "Jeff," I said to my husband after we'd put the kids to bed, "I just can't stand having this stuff in the house anymore."

So we went through our kitchen, looking at the food on our shelves. I had been a devoted Costco shopper; it just made so much sense to me to buy my food there in giant bulk! Now I looked at the gallon-sized tank of bright-orange Goldfish crackers and thought about the genetically modified corn and soy they contained, and rBGH-laden cheese, and all the chemicals that had been added to turn them that glowing color, and my heart sank. I had thought Goldfish were a healthier choice than po-tato chips, but maybe not.

I looked at the super-sized bags of Tostito corn chips in the wooden box on the floor, the one with the hinged top, so my kids could help themselves to snacks. I had thought they were a healthier choice than Doritos or cheese puffs. Now all I could think of were those insecticidal toxins, engineered right into every kernel of corn.

We looked in our pantry. There were rows and rows of blue boxes of Kraft Macaroni & Cheese, a food I remembered fondly from my own childhood. If my mother had thought it was okay to give it to us, why wouldn't I think it was good for my own kids? I never just gave them mac 'n' cheese, I'd always add a green vegetable and maybe an apple or a banana to the plate. But now even that seemed a dereliction of duty as I wondered about the rBGH, the soy, the corn, and the chemicals. And I hated to think of Kraft funding FAAN's Web site, which still refused to discuss any potential link between GM foods and allergies—except, of course, for the post they'd done to refute me.

I looked in our refrigerator. Layered into the freezer were some giant bags of dinosaur-shaped chicken nuggets, another staple. The kids loved them, and I had thought they were healthier than hot dogs and lower in fat than red meat. But they had been made from corn-fed chickens and they, too, probably contained soy filler and perhaps more corn in the breading. And what about the antibiotics that likely lurked in the chicken meat itself?

Jeff and I toured our whole kitchen, and part of me just wanted to throw the whole lot out, just junk it all and start over again. I wanted to give my kids only the healthiest, purest, most perfect foods—foods that I knew for a fact would only be good for them, from now on through their ripe old ages. No hidden allergens, no cancer-causing hormones, no weird-science DNA. Just good healthy food that showed my kids how much I loved them.

But when we finished looking through our cupboards and refrigerator shelves, I knew I couldn't do anything so drastic. For one thing, it wasn't in our budget. Not to mention that the kids would freak out. And besides, what would I feed them? Of course I wished we lived in a world where everything could be pure and perfect. But right now, we lived in *this* world.

That's when I first came up with the 80–20 rule, which I have to say has been a lifesaver, both in terms of our health and in terms of my sanity. I thought, *Maybe I can't be 100 percent pure, but why can't I go for 80 percent?* I could still serve my kids noodles—but maybe I could just use a little portion of the powder, or switch from bright-yellow cheese to the white cheddar variety, or even (though this took me a few more months) just grate some cheese onto those noodles myself. I could still serve them chips, but maybe potato chips that weren't artificially colored. I was not out to make the perfect the enemy of the good—but I had to cope with the real world, which contained my real kids, a limited budget, picky eaters, and no time!

I didn't come to a whole new way of cooking in that one night, and in many ways, I'm still experimenting. (You can read more about the kitchen-coping strategies I came up with in chapter 8, along with the ways Jeff and I worked out to win over our very *anti*-veggie kids.) But that night was a turning point, because I realized both that I had to start somewhere and that I couldn't expect to do everything at once. Maybe I was a type A, overachieving, "do it all" kind of person, but even I had my limits. I had to accept that though I couldn't do everything, I could certainly do *something*. My four kids deserved to have the same value placed on their lives as had been placed on the lives of children around the world.

So I accepted that I had to start somewhere and move slowly. And for me, that realization was a giant leap forward.

6

TRUE COLORS

Back in January 2006, Tory's allergy had hit our family like an explosion: one of those overwhelming events that demands to be noticed and dealt with. But by the spring of 2007, I had realized that she was not the only child in my family with food allergies. Colin's severe reaction to corn had made that clear.

What I didn't realize was that corn wasn't the only thing Colin was allergic to. Nor did I realize how deeply another allergy was affecting his entire five-year-old being. This second bout with a kid's allergy was less like a terrifying explosion and more like a low, menacing hum: I knew something was wrong, but I didn't always know what, or where, or what to do about it.

Colin had always been a quiet, incredibly serious little kid, rarely one to show his emotions or to welcome affection. The other children held out their arms for big good-night hugs and kisses; Colin maybe allowed me to rub noses with him. The other children burst into smiles when they saw me or Jeff; Colin came over immediately when one of us picked him up after school or returned home after an absence, but his face barely changed. The preschool teacher told us that his nickname among the staff was "Conservative Colin," because he always seemed so sober, so literal and restrained.

Colin also struggled with a number of health problems, which my pediatrician, parents, and friends all assured me were part of the normal apparatus of childhood: eczema; a deep, persistent cough; and frequent ear infections. But he'd had so many respiratory infections as an infant that I had been warned by my pediatrician that he'd probably develop asthma. And his eczema was something above and beyond what most kids suffered with. He seemed afflicted with a permanently raw, red rash that covered both his armpits and persisted no matter what over-the-counter or prescription creams I tried. He and I both were pretty mortified about exposing it in public on a hot day or at the pool. By the spring of 2007, we had graduated to a hideously strong steroid-based ointment that made me nervous every time I applied it—what in the world might it be doing to my little boy's hormones?—but which seemed worth a try if it could make the itching and rawness stop and ease the embarrassment that he so obviously felt when exposing his skin in public.

Likewise, Colin's cough seemed more than the usual childhood tickle in the throat. It was a deep, bronchial rattle that sounded—I hate to say it—full of mucus. When he lay down to sleep, he'd sometimes cough for an hour at a time before finally dropping off. And his earaches were so frequent that the pediatrician prescribed ongoing rounds of antibiotics that did nothing to solve the ear infections but that did create some serious gastrointestinal issues, giving my little boy the constant runs.

Finally, the doctor suggested either putting Colin on a daily low dose of antibiotics (which, given what was already happening to his poops, horrified me) or operating on him with ear-tube surgery. We reluctantly chose the latter, though I canceled the procedure twice before finally putting my child under.

It broke my heart to see my son struggle with so many supposedly minor childhood ailments, not to mention how exhausting the sleepless nights and pediatrician's visits had become. The doctor's reassurances that they were normal seemed cold comfort when I thought of how hard they all were on Colin. Thanks to the surgery, the earaches did stop, but the raw, embarrassing rash persisted.

Then in March 2007, Jeff and I took the kids down to a little beach town in Texas to share a vacation with my Houston-based parents. "Oh, Jeff," I said to my husband on the plane. "I can just imagine how feeding the kids organic food is going to go over down here. Everyone's going to think our kids are 'social outcasts with eating disorders' and that I'm some Boulder hippie freak. Do you think it would help if I wore a business suit to the beach?"

Jeff laughed, and so did I, but I was seriously worried about how my new commitment to healthy eating would fit into what I pictured as the conservative Texas where I'd grown up. Imagine my surprise, then, when I walked into the local branch of a national grocery chain and found that 30 percent of the produce section was organic!

I was stunned. I must have stood in front of the lettuce for at least five minutes, just reading the signs. When Jeff came over to join me, I took his hand.

"It wasn't like this when I was growing up," I said, still staring at the organic lettuce. "Something has really changed."

I turned to face him. "Maybe I won't sound so weird, after all. If a small town in Texas has converted this quickly to an organic selection, maybe my ideas won't be viewed as some 'hippie' thing, Maybe other people *are* going to get the message, if I can ever figure out how to get it out there. Maybe, on some level, most people already know that something's wrong, and they'll be ready to hear what I've been finding out."

Jeff, who had grown up in Seattle, wasn't as shocked by the organic section as I was. But when we reached the dairy counter, we were both disappointed to discover that this otherwise well-stocked grocery was out of rBGH-free milk.

Many parents would be distressed to think of depriving their kids of dairy products for a week, especially given the extremely successful "Got Milk?" campaign that has gotten us all convinced that dairy is the way to go. But I was actually less upset about my kids' nutrition than I was about the thought of how Colin and John would respond to going milkless for a week. My two boys guzzled milk the way SUVs guzzle gas. At bedtime alone, Colin drank three glasses a night.

Still, after what I'd learned about rBGH, I just couldn't bring myself to buy regular milk anymore. I looked at the rows of cheerful red-and-white cartons and all I could think of was growth hormones, cancer, and udder pus. "We'll do without milk for one week," I decided. "It won't kill us."

Although Colin and John both clamored for their favorite drink when we returned from the store, we told them that we hadn't bought any and weren't going to, because the grocery store in this new town didn't have the kind of milk we liked. They weren't thrilled with that answer, but between the beach, the grandparents, and the fun of being on vacation, they had more than enough exciting distractions to keep them occupied.

As the week wore on, Jeff and I noticed that Colin's underarm eczema was slowly getting better. For the first time in years, his skin was no longer raw. We put the change down to extra sun and maybe the healing salty beachside air, but I couldn't help hoping that maybe my little boy had somehow outgrown the skin condition that had given him such discomfort. Could we finally breathe a sigh of relief?

No such luck. Within a week of getting him back to Colorado, he was totally rashed out, his armpits as red and raw as they'd ever been. And his cough was back. In fact, it was only after returning to Colorado and hearing that sad, familiar bedtime hacking start up again that Jeff and I realized how much better his cough had been in Texas.

"It was better down there, right?" I asked Jeff. "I kind of didn't notice it, but now that it's come back . . ."

"No, it was better," Jeff agreed.

We looked at each other. I don't remember which one of us said it first: "Do you think it is caused by the milk?"

The math seemed simple enough. No milk, no cough, no eczema. It seemed pretty obvious that we should try to wean Colin away from milk.

Now here is where you'll see what a food purist I am *not*. It honestly didn't even occur to me that Colin should be kept away from *all* dairy products. Our little inadvertent experiment had been restricted to the effects of milk, so it was milk and milk alone that I tried to restrict in Colin's diet. My son went right on eating cheese, yogurt, and prepared foods that included milk, like granola bars with chocolate chips in them. It was only the liquid white stuff that I tried to keep him away from. But given his addiction, this one adjustment alone was a huge one in my little boy's diet.

I'll be honest: the weaning process was not one of the more fun times I've ever had with Colin, who had become so hooked on his nightly cups and daily glasses of milk. In fact, it was worse than when I had weaned him from the bottle. (It was so brutal at points that I actually address the weaning process in chapter 8, where I also offer some step-by-step suggestions on how to wean *your* child from problem foods.)

But somehow, we managed. And to everybody's astonishment and joy, Colin's eczema, cough, and earaches disappeared completely.

One night in the tub, Lexy even commented on it. "Colin, your armpits aren't red and gross anymore."

"Yeah, I know," was all he said. And we all looked at the soft pink scars that remained where the raw, red rash had been.

As Colin drank less milk, though, he began to switch to yogurt. By this time, it was the white kind that I let the kids sweeten by adding their choice of blueberries, raisins, jelly, honey, or on special occasions, colorful sprinkles—no more blue tubes!—so I thought of it as pretty healthy. But when I saw Colin switch from milk-guzzling to yogurt-guzzling, I began to worry. Something in the way he craved dairy products so intensely set off one of those Mama warning bells, where you just feel that something's off.

Around that time, a friend told me about the work of Kenneth Bock, MD, the doctor whose work I've highlighted in earlier chapters, so I ordered his book *Healing the New Childhood Epidemics*. I opened it the afternoon it arrived and, from the first chapter, I was riveted. I literally read it cover to cover standing in the kitchen that night. I could not put it down. It was the story of Colin.

In the book, Dr. Bock describes a milk-allergic person's cravings for milk as a kind of addiction. I now understood that Colin had appeared to be having an actual chemical reaction to casein, one of the ingredients in milk protein. Although the casein produced his symptoms, it also set up a craving not unlike what alcoholics or drug addicts feel for the substances that make *them* sick. At the time, I didn't understand this consciously, but somehow I must have sensed it, because I began the slow, painful process of weaning Colin from yogurt as well.

With neither milk nor yogurt in his system, Colin's personality slowly began to change. He was still a very intense and literal child—I'm sure he'll always be that way—but a sunny, bubbly side to his personality started to emerge as well. After a few weeks on the no-dairy diet, he began to smile. He started letting me give him real bedtime hugs—he even started asking for them. After years of physical distance from my son, I had no idea how good those hugs were going to feel.

Then, that summer, we went to visit Jeff's family in Seattle. Jeff's mom is a *huge* fan of yogurt, which she, like most of us, sees as one of the healthiest foods a person could possibly eat. And for people without a dairy allergy, she's right: servings of low- or nonfat plain yogurt (pus- and rBGH-free, of course!) each week are a great idea. Knowing this, I suspected that Jeff's mom might have a tough time accepting that one of her grandchildren was being kept from this super-healthy and nutritious food, especially since he himself had always loved "Grammy's yogurt."

What could I do? I went back and forth a few times in my head, then I thought, it's just one week. Why pick a battle over a yogurt pot? So I let Grammy feed Colin the three bowls of yogurt he quickly wheedled out of her and settled in to unpacking. And within maybe three hours, Colin was having the temper tantrum of his life.

My poor mother-in-law. And my poor son. I saw him crying, calling his grandmother names, practically bouncing off the walls in pain and frustration, and I realized that all this crazy behavior was because he was in pain and his system was no longer able to process the food that had given him eczema, headaches, stomachaches, the cough, and that eternal earache. Jeff and I looked at each other.

"I guess we've got to get serious about this dairy thing," he said to me under his breath.

I nodded.

The Southampton Shocker

Remember, before my daughter had her first allergic reaction, I was one of those people who rolled their eyes when other parents talked about their kids' sensitivity to this, that, or the other. I had heard moms talk about how little Hannah couldn't tolerate milk products or darling Connor was a beast if they didn't keep his diet clean and pure, and I thought, "Oh, toughen up," or "Maybe try disciplining your kids instead of blaming their bad behavior on the food," or even "Well, that's one way to make your kid the center of the universe—and you, too, while you're at it."

Now *I* had become one of those mothers who insisted that *her* children couldn't have milk, yogurt, or eggs, let alone nonorganic this or processed that, and I winced every time I saw people rolling their eyes at *me*. How I wished I could take back every unsympathetic thought, every misinformed reply, and every judgment I had ever passed!

One good thing that came out of the whole process, though, was that when new scientific evidence emerged on the ways that artificial colors and other additives affected kids' behavior, I looked at this information with a new understanding. Although mainstream scientists had for years pooh-poohed the idea that diet could have a significant effect on children with attention-deficit hyperactivity disorder (ADHD), a study coming out of the University of Southampton in the U.K. turned that opinion around. In September 2007, a research team from the University of Southampton's Schools of Psychology and Medicine shocked much of the conventional medical world with their dramatic findings about the effects on children of artificial colors and preservatives.

Throughout the late 1980s and 1990s, a handful of previous studies had been conducted into the effects of artificial colors and/or preservatives on kids who had—or behaved as though they had—ADHD. I was also aware of the Feingold Association, a group of families and professionals dedicated to promoting the dietary approach of allergist Ben F. Feingold, MD, which had been around since 1976. Their food plan consisted of eliminating artificial coloring (of initial concern to Feingold's team in part because these artificial colors were derived from petroleum), synthetic flavoring, aspartame (sold as NutraSweet and Equal artificial sweeteners), and artificial preservatives. This diet was originally designed as a diet for children with allergies, but an improvement in behavior and attention was eventually noticed—as a side effect!

Nevertheless, mainstream medical and scientific opinion remained unconvinced. Then came the unusually large and well-received 2007 study, the one that I came to think of as the Southampton Shocker.

Researchers at Southampton University studied 153 three-year-olds and 144 eight-year-olds, a strikingly large number for research of this kind. Because it's so hard to find enough families able to participate in long-term dietary studies, which involve huge, dramatic changes in children's eating habits, many previous studies had counted their subjects not in the hundreds but in the dozens. The breadth of the Southampton study and the dramatic nature of its findings went a long way toward convincing many who had previously been skeptics. It also helped that the study was published in an online edition of *The Lancet,* one of the world's most prestigious medical journals, the U.K. equivalent of the *New England Journal of Medicine.*

The children in the study were chosen from the general residential population of Southampton, England, and they represented the full spectrum of childhood behavior, from normal through hyperactive. For six weeks, the kids were given a diet free from the additives the study was focusing on. The kids were also given something to drink each day: One group got a mix of artificial colors (the kinds found in candy, bright-orange mac 'n' cheese, and even kids' medicines and vitamins) and the preservative sodium benzoate (used in most sodas and soft drinks). The other group got a "neutral" drink, also known as a *placebo,* a substance that has no physical effect.

The real drink and the placebo looked and tasted exactly the same, so the children and their families had no idea which drink the kids were given. Even the researchers who handed out the drinks didn't know, so that their attitudes wouldn't affect the families' responses. (This is known as a *double-blind study,* in which neither subjects nor researchers know who gets the "real stuff" and who gets the placebo. That way, scientists can be sure that they're observing actual results and not the psychological responses of people who *believe* they're being helped.)

After the children were given the drinks, their behavior was described by their parents and teachers, as well as by an observer from the study who watched them at school. The older kids also got a computer-based test of their attention.

The results were strikingly clear. Children who consumed the mix of food coloring and the sodium benzoate demonstrated marked behavioral changes. They were significantly more hyperactive: they moved more, they were more impulsive, and they had trouble keeping their attention on a particular topic.

The research team was led by psychology professor Jim Stevenson, who asserted that the study provided "clear evidence that mixtures of certain food colours and benzoate preservative can adversely influence the behaviour of children."

Stevenson was quick to add a note of caution. "[P]arents should not think that simply taking these additives out of food will prevent all hyperactive disorders," he said. "We know that many other influences are at work, but this at least is one a child can avoid."

I was fascinated to read the Southampton study when it came out, because I knew that the question of diet, behavior, and ADHD had been hotly debated for quite a while. A number of previous studies had suggested a correlation. As early as April 24, 1988, an edition of the *Australian Paediatric Journal* had published the results of a study of 220 children believed to be hyperactive.

Of this initial group, fifty-five were given a six-week trial of the Feingold diet, the one without additives, preservatives, artificial colors, or aspartame. Almost three-quarters of the children showed "improved behavior" during the diet, and about half "remained improved" even after the diet was liberalized during the following three to six months.

Parents of fourteen of the children said that certain types of behaviors seemed to result when their kids ate artificial or synthetically colored foods, so researchers conducted a double-blind study with eight of these children, giving them either a placebo or one of two types of artificial color, tartrazine (which dyes foods bright yellow and is also known as FD&C Yellow 5) or carmoisine (which dyes foods bright red). Two of the children who were given the dyes showed extreme irritability, restlessness, and sleep disturbance—reactions that seemed to be a response to the additives.

True, this was a very small study. And only two out of the eight children given the dyes reacted. But those children reacted very strongly, with behaviors that otherwise might have been attributed either to their ADHD or to their personalities. And that's one out of every four kids. Could that be my angelic, mischievous, hyper John?

So here is where I'll admit to reacting as a parent, rather than as a skeptic. My Research Wonk side looks at the Australian study and says, "Hey, if only eight children were studied and only two children reacted, that's really not enough data to let us draw conclusions. Yeah, two out of eight constitutes 25 percent, but let's wait until someone does a bigger study before we start applying these statistics and telling parents to change their kids' diets."

But the mom in me says, "*What?* You mean that this might affect one of *my* four kids and there's a chance that changing my kid's diet means he'll be less cranky, better behaved, and more likely to sleep better? I get that this won't necessarily work on all kids, and that the results are more dramatic with some kids than with others—fine! But if there's *any* chance at all with *my* kid, maybe we should give this diet thing a try."

I looked at my kids. Since they had been unwitting guinea pigs in the live human trial that Monsanto was apparently conducting on all of us, with their genetically engineered milk, corn, and soy, could I engage them in my own Southampton study in suburbia? As with Colin and the milk, I just might try to do my own study. (And if you want to try your own study in cutting back the additives, check out chapter 8 for some easy-to-follow suggestions.)

Colorful Research

If the tiny Australian study were the only precursor to the Southampton
Shocker, I might still have remained skeptical. But as I started to look
into the matter, I discovered that more research had revealed the beneficial effects of diet—though interestingly, none of these positive findings
were being found in the United States. For example, a 1993 British study
published in the *Archives of Disease in Childhood* concerned seventy-
eight children referred to a diet clinic because of their hyperactive behavior. These kids were put on a highly restricted diet, given only a few
"neutral" foods with no sugar, additives, or preservatives. During this period, almost three fourths of the children—fifty-nine, to be exact—improved in behavior.

Then, after having been observed on a relatively "clean" diet, some
nineteen children were given disguised "problem foods" and/or additives
(some were given neutral foods, so the scientists would have a basis for
comparison). In other words, the researchers did a proper laboratory version of our own milk experiment with Colin: take the questionable food
out of his diet, see what happens, and then see what happens when you
put it back in.

As with Colin and yogurt, the results were dramatic. Scientists found
"a significant effect for the provoking foods to worsen ratings of behaviour and to impair psychological test performance." Significantly, the
study concluded, *"Clinicians should give weight to the accounts of parents*
and consider this treatment in selected children with a suggestive medical history" (emphasis added).

Wow. So the researchers were admitting that parents who lived with
their children day in and day out might observe behavioral changes that
doctors didn't notice and couldn't always test for. As a mom who had
done a "home experiment" of her own, I appreciated the acknowledgment.

I also thought about what I had learned from Dr. Bock about delayed
sensitivities to foods. Could this explain the difference between what

the scientists observed in the experiments and what parents observed a few days later at home?

But there was more. Tartrazine, a.k.a. E102 or FD&C Yellow 5, which I had learned was found in boxes of mac 'n' cheese in the United States, had been studied by Australian researchers in 1994, who discovered that it affected children's sleep, mood, and behavior.

Published in the *Australian Paediatric Journal,* the study concerned some 200 children in Melbourne, out of a group of about 800 referred to the Royal Children's Hospital there for suspected hyperactivity. For six weeks, the 200 children were given a synthetic-color-free diet—and the parents of 150 of them reported "behavioral improvement." As in the other experiments, parents also noticed "deterioration" of behavior after the kids started eating synthetically colored foods again.

Not entirely satisfied with this general finding, the researchers designed a more precise trial. They selected 34 children aged two to fourteen years, including 23 suspected of reacting to artificial coloring and 11 "uncertain reactors," along with a control group of 20 kids who were believed not to react to coloring at all. They conducted a twenty-one-day double-blind study—again, no one knew who was getting the chemicals and who was getting the placebo—in which each morning a child got either a placebo or one of six dose levels of tartrazine (1, 2, 5, 10, 20, and 50 mg). At the end of each day, parents rated their children. In other words, parents rated their kids' behavior without knowing whether they'd had chemicals that day or not.

The results once again suggested that synthetic colors had a significant effect on behavior. Some 19 of the 23 "suspected reactors," 3 of the 11 "uncertain reactors," and even 2 of the 20 "control group kids"—children previously believed not to react at all—were irritable and restless and had trouble sleeping after being dosed with the yellow dye. Kids reacted at all six dose levels, but when the doses were higher than 10 mg, the effects seemed to last longer.

So, I thought when I read this study, if kids have been loaded up with synthetic colors, it might take a while for their systems to get clean. Keeping our kids on high levels of tartrazine seems to be setting them up for long-term irritability, restlessness, and sleep problems. And even when we take the synthetic colors out of our kids' diet, it may take a while before we see an improvement.

A Brazilian study conducted in 2007 suggested that tartrazine could also cause serious health problems in rats, elevating white blood cells called eosinophils in the gastrointestinal tract. Eosinophils are immune-system white blood cells that destroy parasitic organisms—their "good-cop" function—but also play a major role in provoking allergic reactions—their "bad-cop" function. This seemed like a problem to me! Not to mention that elevated levels of eosinophils in the digestive system and associated lymph nodes may result in nausea, difficulty swallowing, abdominal pain, vomiting, diarrhea, excessive loss of proteins in the gastrointestinal tract, and failure to thrive.

Other studies piled on the data. An earlier Spanish study, dating back to 1981, pointed out that "allergic reactions to food colors have been known since 1958," adding that such colors might be found in a number of prescription drugs that did not even list these ingredients on their labels. A similar Canadian study, also from 1981, found that "from 4% to 14% of individuals with asthma or allergies or both and from 7% to 20% of persons who are sensitive to acetylsalicylic acid [the basic ingredient in aspirin] may react to [tartrazine]," adding a recommendation that tartrazine content appear on drug labels. (So far, it doesn't.)

The Southampton folks had also done a previous study in 2004, also published in the *Archives of Disease in Childhood*. This earlier Southampton study concerned some 1,873 three-year-olds from the general population and, like the later study, was intended to determine whether artificial colorings and/or preservatives affected hyperactive behavior. (Almost two thousand three-year-olds!—can you imagine?)

As in the other studies, the kids were given a special diet with no artificial colors or benzoate-based preservatives. They got this restricted diet for only one week, which was probably a lot easier for the scientists and parents to administer, though as the Australian study suggested—and as many parents will attest—some kids take more time to show results.

Then, for the next three weeks, the children got either a drink full of colors and sodium benzoate or a placebo. Again, this was a *double-blind study:* neither researchers, parents, nor kids knew who was getting the neutral drink and who was getting the chemical cocktail. But all the kids in the study got some of both—some weeks, they got chemicals, some weeks they were preservative- and color-free.

The results were, once again, dramatic. In the words of the study, "There were significant reductions in hyperactive behaviour" during the time when kids were taken off the chemicals and "significantly greater increases in hyperactive behaviour" during the weeks that kids *were* getting chemicals.

Remember, parents had no idea which weeks their kids had gotten the chemicals and which weeks they'd gotten the placebo. Even the researchers handing out the drinks didn't know. But the parental reports— the basis of this earlier Southampton study—were very clear. During the chemical-free weeks, kids were relatively well behaved. During the chemical cocktail weeks, they were hyper.

Again, I want to share with you the exact wording of the study's conclusion: "There is a general adverse effect of artificial food colouring and benzoate preservatives on the behaviour of 3 year old children *which is detectable by parents* but *not* by a simple clinic assessment."

I added the emphasis because I want everyone to hear those words loud and clear. The scientists themselves were saying that parents, who live with their children day in and day out, often notice dietary effects that doctors miss. Now, how many of us have had the experience of telling a doctor how this or that food seems to affect our kid, only to be told that there's no scientific evidence for the effect we're noticing? I had to wonder why the doctors in the United States weren't as open-minded and respectful of parents' judgments as their counterparts in Great Britain.

Finally, an Australian study published in the May 24, 2008, edition of the *British Medical Journal* followed up the Southampton Shocker with another double-blind study of 297 children aged three to nine years, none of whom had ever been diagnosed with ADHD. Yet even these "normal" children, when given a mix of synthetic colors and sodium benzoate that "approximated that found in two 56 gram bags of sweets" (or about two two-ounce bags of candy), displayed increased hyperactive behavior. Only four ounces of candy caused "normal" children to react! If that wasn't scientific validation for what every parent already suspects, I don't know what is.

Think for a moment about what it might mean to take these "hyper" additives out of our kids' diets. Even if cutting out artificial colors and sodium benzoate by just four ounces means that your kids are only getting, say, another twenty minutes' sleep each night because they are less hyper and agitated, think about how that adds up. Initially, it might just allow you to breathe a sigh of relief when bedtime comes. But think about what it might do for your kids: an extra twenty minutes of sleep each night turns into almost two and a half hours more of sleep each week. And then that turns into an extra ten hours of sleep a month. Who knows what effects that additional sleep time might have on your children's mood (and yours!), let alone on their alertness, problem-solving abilities, and school performance. And think about how the teachers would benefit if they were to have an entire classroom of first-graders getting a few extra winks a night.

New research out of the University of Berkeley and elsewhere demonstrates that most children need far more sleep than they're currently getting and that sleep is far more crucial to their intelligence, mood, and overall well-being than we'd ever suspected. Certainly, there are lots of factors involved in children's sleep habits, including time spent in front of a TV or computer screen: the flickering electronic light stimulates wakefulness (that's true for adults, too!). Clearly, too, children's hyperactive behavior has many sources, as does crankiness and other behavioral problems.

But if standing on a thumbtack hurts, you get off of the thumbtack! You don't take aspirin until it stops hurting! The same logic applies here. If consuming chemicals keeps you hyper and active, doesn't it make sense to eliminate the chemicals?

It also seems clear that some children are far more affected by artificial colors and preservatives than others. When Massachusetts General Hospital's Thomas Spencer, MD, was asked to comment on the 2007 Southampton Shocker, the one of all these studies that finally made headlines here in the United States, he told the *New York Times* that some children may be " 'supersensitive to additives' just as some people are more sensitive to caffeine."

In other words, some children may be "supersensitive," while others, presumably, aren't much affected. Okay. But if your child is one of the "supersensitive" ones, wouldn't you like to know that changing his or her diet, even just a little bit, might make a world of difference? I like the comparison to caffeine, because I can see the differences in my own family: my mom can drink coffee all day long and still sleep soundly at night, while I can barely tolerate two cups a day and only before 6 p.m.

It's that way with allergies, too: my girls can apparently consume colors, no problem, while those particular chemicals seem to turn John and Colin from sunny Dr. Jekylls into nightmarish Mr. Hydes!

So, clearly, we don't all need the same diets and we don't all react badly to the same things. If your kids can tolerate bright-yellow food coloring and sodium benzoate, maybe you don't need to worry quite so much about changing that part of their diets. But until you cut back on the chemicals, even by as little as four ounces, you may never know just how much their so-called normal childhood difficulties are being intensified or even created by what they're eating. Think about that during the next bedtime battle or after-school tantrum, and maybe a chemical-reduction experiment won't sound quite so crazy. (For some ideas on how to *easily* and *gradually* reduce your kids' chemical intake, see chapter 8.)

How Sweet It Isn't: The Aspartame Analysis

Artificial colors are everywhere, it seems. But so is the artificial sweetener aspartame—the basis for NutraSweet and Equal—which is used in everything from Diet Coke to Yoplait yogurt. And since it was one of the

chemical additives that continued to be mentioned in association with
the Southampton Shocker study, I decided to take a look.

Well, if there was a small flurry of studies on synthetic coloring, the
research done on aspartame qualifies as a huge blizzard. Aspartame has
been linked to a host of deadly diseases, including brain tumors, brain lesions, and lymphoma. Meanwhile, the story of how this controversial
substance came to be approved by the FDA reads like a John Grisham
novel, with a cast of government and corporate figures that includes Donald Rumsfeld and the Monsanto Corporation. If you want to understand
both the science and the politics of synthetic ingredients, aspartame of-
fers almost a classic example of what can go wrong with both.

The story of aspartame begins in 1981, when the substance was first
approved by the FDA as an artificial sweetener for human consumption.
Fourteen years later, in 1995, the chief of the FDA's Epidemiology
Branch—the division that monitors the incidence of diseases and medical problems—reported that in those fourteen years, complaints about
aspartame constituted 75 percent of all FDA reports concerning adverse
reactions to food.

Wow. Seventy-five percent of all complaints. Wouldn't you think a
number like that would give the FDA pause, maybe make it reconsider
its approval?

Of course, just because someone reports a complaint doesn't mean
the complaint is justified. Either a patient or a doctor might believe, in-
correctly, that aspartame caused a condition that was actually caused by
something else. Still—75 percent? That's a *lot* of aspartame-related complaints: three times as many as all the other complaints put together.

But let's not rely on people's (and doctors') reports. Let's take a look at
the scientific research that has been done.

First, though, I should tell you that the possible harmful effects of aspartame is one of the most hotly contested topics you could possibly find
in the field of nutrition. Some human and animal studies have shown
disastrously adverse effects, while others have shown that the artificial
sweetener is just fine. As prestigious a scientist as David Ludwig, MD,
the Harvard researcher working with obese children whom we met in

chapter 2, believes that when you consider the adverse effects of obesity, aspartame is definitely the lesser of two evils.

If I cite every pro and con aspartame study that's come out in the past fifteen years, I could fill a whole other book, so let me just mention a few conditions that aspartame has been accused of causing:

BRAIN TUMORS In November 1996, the *Journal of Neuropathology and Experimental Neurology* published a scientific paper saying that aspartame might be responsible for a dramatic increase in the number of people who develop brain tumors. Reported in a CBS News/60 *Minutes* broadcast, the Swedish study found a link among elderly and middle-aged people between drinking diet sodas and developing certain types of large brain tumors.

MEMORY LAPSES A 2001 *Psychology Today* article reported on a Texas Christian University study suggesting that aspartame users were more likely to report long-term memory lapses. "After reporting his findings at a recent Society for Neuroscience meeting," the article continued, "[psychology professor Timothy M.] Barth [PhD] cautioned that he thinks it's premature to condemn aspartame. But he does worry about the largely untested effects of long-term use."

WEIGHT GAIN A 1997 study at the University of Texas Health Sciences Center, reported at a meeting of the American Diabetes Association, found a "41 percent increase in the risk of being overweight for every can or bottle of diet soft drink a person consumes each day." These findings were supported by another study, published in the *Journal of Applied Nutrition,* showing that 5 percent of subjects who reported symptoms from aspartame also reported a "paradoxic weight gain." And a study in the *International Journal of Obesity* likewise found that women who were dieting tended to take in more calories after consuming aspartame than after ingesting either sugar or water.

LYMPHOMAS, LEUKEMIA, AND OTHER CANCERS A long-term Italian study conducted by Italy's Ramazzini Foundation by Morando Soffritti and his colleagues and published in the summer of 2005 in the *European Journal of Oncology* linked aspartame to lymphomas and leukemias in animals. A 2005 follow-up study published in *Environmental Health Per-*

spectives showed that aspartame was linked to a significant increase in cancer of the kidney and peripheral nerves.

This Italian study has also been the subject of controversy. Both the European Food Safety Authority (EFSA) and our own FDA concluded that these findings were not cause for concern. The FDA claimed to have found "significant shortcomings" in the Italian study, shortcomings that "compromised" its findings. In August 2007, the New Zealand Food Safety Authority concurred, issuing a press release criticizing the study and affirming the safety of aspartame.

Further criticism of the Italian study came, implicitly, from the National Cancer Institute (NCI), which published a study in April 2006 finding no meaningful link between aspartame and leukemia, lymphoma, or brain tumor. The study relied on 1995 and 1996 surveys completed by 340,045 men and 226,945 women—obviously, a huge number—detailing what they ate and drank. Based on follow-up data from this sample, the NCI concluded, you couldn't link aspartame and cancer.

However, the NCI study also had its critics, who pointed out that the Italian study was designed to measure *lifelong* consumption of aspartame, focusing on its cumulative effects, rather than considering only a few years. Moreover, the humans in the NCI study were middle-aged, whereas, according to neurosurgeon Dr. Russell Blaylock, "The greatest risk of leukemia and lymphoma would be in a younger population (young children and adolescents) and they would need to be exposed regularly from early in life."

Clearly, this is a case where the experts would appear to disagree. If even the scientists can't agree on whether aspartame is safe or not, how are we mere mortals supposed to decide?

Well, remember my ethics professor, the one who told me always to look at who benefits? So who benefits from saying aspartame is safe? The aspartame industry. And guess what? An analysis of peer-reviewed medical literature conducted by Ralph G. Walton, MD and cited in a CBS News/60 *Minutes* segment that aired in December 1996 found that of the studies in the review, 100 percent of those funded by the aspartame industry had found that aspartame was safe.

Hmmm. What about the *non*-industry-funded studies? Dr. Walton's analysis found that of the ninety non-industry-funded studies, eighty-two of them, or a whopping 92 percent, identified one or more problems with aspartame. And of the seven which found aspartame innocuous, six were conducted by the FDA, an agency which, as we saw in chapter 4 and as we'll see later in this chapter, has virtually installed its own revolving door to welcome past and future executives from the food industry.

I find this information so shocking that I'm going to repeat it, just in case you think you might have read it wrong: *All* the industry-funded studies said aspartame was completely safe. *Ninety-two percent* of the independent studies said aspartame poses at least some dangers (99 percent if you don't count studies conducted by the industry-riddled FDA).

Who do *you* think has the greatest incentive to tell the truth?

If you need one more piece of evidence to make you doubt industry-funded research, let me cite one last study, concerning medical articles about soft drinks, juice, and milk. A team of researchers, including Harvard's David Ludwig (mentioned above and in chapter 2), as well as other researchers from Children's Hospital in Boston and the Center for Science in the Public Interest in Washington, D.C., reviewed 206 articles published during 1999–2003. Of these articles, 111 disclosed financial sponsorship: 22 percent were entirely funded by the food industry; 47 percent had no industry ties; and 32 percent had mixed funding. Doesn't that make you wonder about why *all* studies don't disclose their financial sponsorship?

The researchers concluded, "Funding source was significantly related to conclusions when considering all article types. . . . Industry funding of nutrition-related scientific articles may bias conclusions in favor of sponsors' products, with potentially significant implications for public health."

In other words, when industry pays for a study, it tends to get science that supports the safety of its products. And when a study is independently funded—as with the ninety aspartame studies Dr. Walton analyzed—it is far more likely (in the case of aspartame, 92 percent more likely) to be critical of a food, a drink, or an additive, with, as Dr. Ludwig at Harvard had just pointed out, "potentially significant implications for public health."

Above and beyond the funding, other scientists have raised questions both about the substance and about the research that's been done to investigate it. A 1998 Spanish study conducted on rats found that aspartame ultimately converts to formaldehyde in the body, and then tends to accumulate in the brain, liver, kidneys, and other tissues. Industry scientists, however, replied that the Spanish scientists weren't actually measuring formaldehyde, but rather some other by-products from aspartame, which perhaps are not as harmful.

So if someone tells you that there's still a lot of controversy about aspartame, technically, they're right. But when you hear people arguing over whether the product is safe, be aware that the ones who say it is tend to be either from the food or chemical industries or from government agencies that fill key positions with food industry executives and sometimes even corporate shareholders.

The independent scientists, on the other hand, insist that aspartame is dangerous—and they've been doing so for more than forty years. When it comes to my health and the health of my kids, I think I'll listen to them.

The Aspartame Affair

As if the potential dangers of aspartame weren't scary enough, the story of how this sweetener came to win FDA approval is the stuff of nightmares—or at least, in the fall of 2006 when I first learned about it, it was the stuff of *my* nightmares.

The aspartame story really hit me where I lived because, not only did I grow up drinking diet sodas, but as I've already said, I began this whole journey as a quiet conservative, a business major, and a sincere supporter of our system. As a matter of fact, to share how personally affected I was by my next discovery, I must disclose that I was also a lifelong Republican. So in the fall of 2006, the idea of our Republican leaders helping corporations win approval for a potentially harmful substance was beyond my comprehension. When I share this story with you, perhaps you'll be as shocked as I was—or then again, maybe you won't. But for me, it shattered my world.

The story was first told by the United Press International (UPI) investigative reporter Gregory Gordon, who spent eight months researching aspartame and then published a three-part series in 1987. The tale begins with the chemical company known as G.D. Searle, which began to study the artificial sweetener in the mid-1960s.

Naturally, Searle wanted to win FDA approval of its chemical sweetener (which we now know as NutraSweet and Equal). Nothing wrong with that! But when you read the internal memos that Gordon dug up, you get the distinct feeling that the company had a few hands at play when it came to their dealings with the government agency: those that were on the table . . . and those beneath.

Now I haven't been living under a rock. I know that industry has remarkable influence over government regulations. After all, that is what our lobbying system is designed to do! But when I began reading these internal memos, I was struck by the sense of ownership that Searle and its executives appeared to exhibit over the FDA.

"We must create an affirmative atmosphere in our dealing with them," wrote Searle official Herbert Helling in a December 28, 1970, memo to Searle senior company executives, suggesting that the company create proposals carefully in order to put FDA officials "into a yes saying habit" and "help bring them into a subconscious spirit of participation."

Helling got what he wanted. On July 26, 1974, only fifteen months after Searle first made its request, FDA commissioner Alexander Schmidt approved aspartame for use in dry foods, despite the apparent risks associated with the chemical.

FDA commissioner Schmidt only allowed thirty days for comments on his ruling, a time frame that outraged consumer groups and neuropathologist Dr. John Olney of Washington University, who had linked aspartame to brain lesions in mice. So Schmidt froze the approval and, in a first-ever action, ordered the creation of a public board of inquiry to investigate the artificial sweetener.

This move was not entirely unfounded given that Searle was also under fire for some of its pharmaceuticals. Ultimately, the investigative team was expected to review the scientific studies that Searle had used to win approval for five of its drugs and for its Copper-7 intrauterine device. However, upon completing the review, the FDA team excoriated the company's poor research methods and wrote that the FDA could not rely upon the firm's integrity.

Reading the list of Searle's distortions has a kind of Frankenstein's-laboratory feel. The task force accused the company of removing tumors from live animals, for example, to cover up the possibility that their products caused cancer. The company was also accused of storing animal tissues in formaldehyde until they deteriorated—presumably, so that they could not be studied. Although a group of monkeys had apparently suffered seizures after being fed aspartame, Searle scientists decided not to autopsy them. Instead, the company paid for a new monkey study that used a different approach to test the sweetener—and *those* monkeys showed no problems.

As I read this, all I could think of was aspartame's 100 percent safety record in those studies funded by the aspartame industry. Is this how it was achieved?

The FDA even asked the U.S. attorney's office to open a grand jury investigation of the company. So Searle spent seven years waiting for aspartame to be approved, while the task force's findings were sorted out.

Then a new character entered the story—a new character whose name was shockingly familiar. In 1977, the Searle company named as its new president a man named Donald Rumsfeld.

When I got to this part of the UPI article, I froze. This could not possibly be *the* Donald Rumsfeld, the one that my family had always joked looked like my dad. What in the world was *my* secretary of defense doing running a chemical company?

And as I turned the page, I too entered a revolving door that made the rBGH shenanigans at the FDA look like kids' play—a revolving door so powerful that it spun my belief system into complete disarray. Rumsfeld, Searle, and the FDA united in a series of maneuvers intended to win approval for an artificial sweetener that several scientists had considered potentially unsafe.

First, as Rumsfeld stepped into his leadership role as Searle CEO, Chicago U.S. attorney Samuel Skinner, a Republican appointee, was investigating Searle's drugs and had agreed to meet with Searle's law firm. A month later, Skinner—who was looking to leave office after the election of Democratic president Jimmy Carter—wrote his government aides a memo. Apparently he was considering a job with the very law firm he had just met with—the one representing Searle. And so Skinner withdrew from the Searle matter, delaying the investigation until his designated successor could handle the case.

By the time Skinner's successor took office, only twelve weeks remained before the statute of limitations ran out on allegedly false statements that Searle had made about aspartame. As it happened, the grand jury didn't bring any indictments because those allegations were never explored. The grand jury was convened by Assistant U.S. Attorney William Conlon, who also left the U.S. Attorney's Office fifteen months later to join Searle's law firm.

The Searle story continued with delays, undisclosed information, and apparent efforts to tone down unfavorable findings. The one constant was that old revolving door between the aspartame industry and government, which continued to turn with depressing regularity.

For example, in October 1978, one year after ordering an FDA review that "helped get Searle's petition back on track," according to Gordon's UPI article, FDA official Dr. Howard Roberts left his government post to serve as vice president of the National Soft Drink Association, whose members later marketed diet sodas sweetened with—you guessed it—aspartame. And between 1979 and 1982, writes Gordon, "four more FDA officials who participated in the approval process took jobs linked to the NutraSweet industry."

Somehow, despite all of this industry influence, on September 30, 1980, the FDA's Board of Inquiry ruled against the approval of aspartame. What had those scientists really seen? But Searle was not to be stopped for long.

One month later, in November 1980, Ronald Reagan defeated Jimmy Carter. And though I was only nine at the time, I still remember the air of celebration in our house, where the Reagans had an almost royal status. To watch the president dance, squiring Nancy in her red dress, gave me the feeling, as a child, that I was watching some magnificent combination of Frank Sinatra and a foreign prince with his graceful companion on his arm.

My family was not the only one who was delighted by President Reagan's victory. So, apparently, were Donald Rumsfeld and Searle. And even though Searle was eager to get aspartame on the market, they waited to ask for a reversal until January 21, 1981, the day after Ronald Reagan was sworn into the office of the president.

As I learned this, I felt literally sick to my stomach. Did politics play *that* big a role at the FDA? As a former chief of staff in Republican administrations, did Rumsfeld really wield *that* much influence? Could the food industry really be so powerful?

Of course, the day that Reagan was sworn into office, the Carter-appointed FDA commissioner was still on the job, though he could expect to be replaced fairly soon. But before he left, he set up a special team of scientists with no previous involvement in the issue to review Searle's appeal. Like the other scientists who had looked into the artificial sweetener, this team was also disturbed by the research showing aspartame's potential dangers. Three of the five team members expressed concern, and team member Satya Dubey even wrote an internal memo citing evidence that aspartame might cause brain tumors in rats.

As always happens with new administrations, the old FDA commissioner resigned and the new president appointed his replacement, Arthur Hull Hayes, Jr. And on July 18, 1981, after less than three months in office, the new commissioner ignored his team's response and overturned the board's old ruling. Aspartame, whose approval had been rejected under the previous administration based on scientific evidence that showed it to cause seizures and brain tumors in animals, was now approved for use in dry foods.

Through it all, of course, the revolving door continued to turn. Notably, Hayes eventually resigned amid accusations that he'd accepted gifts from FDA-regulated companies, including General Foods Corporation.

Like most ex–government officials, Hayes went on to a prestigious job—in his case, as dean of the New York Medical School. But he also landed a consulting gig at the New York PR firm Burson-Marsteller—which represented Monsanto. During this period, Monsanto—the company that gave us rBGH and genetically engineered crops—also bought the NutraSweet company, enabling Rumsfeld to profit off of his remarkable regulatory success with aspartame. Just how many connections to the NutraSweet industry did these guys have?

As Searle's CEO, Donald Rumsfeld was now free to market and sell his product. As it happens, aspartame's prime competitor at the time, saccharine, was being widely accused of potentially causing cancer. So, according to Gordon's UPI article, the FDA had just handed Searle "a financial bonanza" in the form of a huge market opportunity for their new product.

According to former Searle sales agent Patty Wood-Allott, Rumsfeld had told his sales force that "he would call in his markers and that no matter what, he would see to it that aspartame would be approved that year."

Of course, we only have Wood-Allott's word for that. But when you look at the evidence—the way Searle waited to appeal until after Reagan took office, and the way the new Reagan-appointed FDA commissioner ignored his team's recommendations and quickly approved Searle's request—it becomes hard *not* to imagine that political connections were somehow involved.

I must admit, when I discovered Donald Rumsfeld's involvement in the approval of aspartame, a product that seemed to pose such a clear potential danger to our health, it shook me to my core. I know that many of you reading this book are now rolling your eyes at *me*! But in the winter of 2006 when I learned this, I didn't understand how the country I loved could operate in such a fashion, and it just flattened me. I didn't see how, if the corruption extended that far, there could be any hope of change. The scope of the food politics that I was up against had been fully exposed.

I took the news personally in another way, too. When I first learned this story, Rumsfeld was still secretary of defense, one of the president's most trusted and influential advisors. As I said in the Introduction, I had been raised on capitalism and the *Wall Street Journal,* and I was *not* looking to call this out. But when I put my kids to bed that night, I realized that that was exactly what I was going to have to do if I was to live with myself. I could not *un*learn what I now knew.

If someone so powerful was working to promote aspartame and to cover up its possible dangers, what hope did I have that anyone would *ever* listen to me? At that point, all I really wanted to do was crawl into a cave and run away from all of this horrible information.

Then I learned how parents in Great Britain had responded to news of the Southampton Shocker—how this one critical study had had such an impact on people's attitudes. I learned, too, how quickly and thoroughly corporations—including the British branches of U.S. companies—had responded to consumer awareness. I realized that ordinary parents and concerned citizens *could* make a difference. And I began to feel hopeful once more.

Corporate Responsibility—U.K. Style

As we've already seen, European countries have often acted before our own government to protect their citizens' health. In Norway, for example, Yellow 5, a.k.a. tartrazine, is banned.

As of this writing tartrazine is *not* federally banned in England. Nevertheless, a whole host of companies, including the U.K. branches of

Wal-Mart, Kraft, Coca-Cola, and the Mars candy company (who make M&M's), have *voluntarily* removed artificial colors, the preservative sodium benzoate, and even Rumsfeld's aspartame from their products.

When I read about this in the spring of 2007, I was stunned. Our American companies had removed these harmful ingredients from their products overseas—but not here? It was one of those stories that I went around repeating to everyone I knew. (My poor friends—they must have been so sick of hearing me talk about food!)

"They've eliminated those additives in England," I kept saying. "Kraft, Mars, and Wal-Mart just took them out." The companies didn't fall apart. The world didn't come to an end. The mums and dads of England weren't condemned to a lifetime of bean sprouts and home-ground oatmeal. They just got to buy mac 'n' cheese and diet colas and grocery-store muffins and even Skittles without the additives that had been shown to make some kids hyper.

So it *was* possible. We *could* have our aspartame-free cake and eat it, too. And we weren't asking anyone to reinvent the wheel. It *was* possible for giant corporations to make and sell kid-friendly, family-friendly, and healthy processed foods. It *was* possible for folks to stroll down the grocery aisles without feeling as though every brightly colored box were a loaded weapon. It was even possible to give your kids some special treats—like the U.K. versions of Starburst and Skittles, for example—without necessarily exposing them to a chemical cocktail that might also give them brain tumors, or leukemia, or the symptoms of ADHD.

When I read the press releases and articles about this breakthrough, I kept being astonished at how far the companies had gone and how quickly they had acted. Asda, for example, the U.K. branch of Wal-Mart—Wal-Mart!—acted just one week "after details were leaked to the UK press of a study by researchers at Southampton University."

Leaked to the press? They didn't even wait for the study to be published—*that's* how concerned they were about public opinion. In Great Britain.

In an article published by the Food and Drink Federation, a Web site that monitors food issues in Europe, Jess Halliday reported that "Asda has pledged to remove any artificial colours or flavours from its 9,000 own label products, as well as aspartame, hydrogenated fat, and flavour enhancers such as monosodium glutamate."

Wow. The Southampton study didn't even mention those last three items. Why was the U.K. Wal-Mart rushing to make such healthy choices, when the U.S. Wal-Mart still offered the same old stuff? Wal-Mart had even been slapped by a lawsuit from Ajinomoto, the company that now makes aspartame, which claimed that U.K. Wal-Mart's publicizing of its aspartame-free products was a kind of defamation—all while the U.S. Wal-Mart continued to use the sweetener.

Even though he had nothing to do with Wal-Mart, I couldn't help but think of Rumsfeld's influence. So if he wasn't the one lobbying the FDA this time, who was?

"[U.K. Wal-Mart] will also meet the Food Standards Agency's salt-reduction targets—two years ahead of the 2010 deadline," the article continued.

Again, wow. Here in the U.S., companies kick and scream and protest FDA rulings and eventually manage to get them overturned. (I am not saying Wal-Mart has done that, but it does seem like a pattern!) But over in England, companies rush to meet government standards two whole years before they even go into effect. And again, why?

According to Asda/U.K. Wal-Mart food trading director Darren Blackhurt, "We know that our customers, particularly those that are mums and dads, are becoming more and more concerned about what's in the food they buy." Indeed, the article continues, "consumer awareness of nutrition and food quality in the UK has soared in the last few years." Accordingly, U.K. Wal-Mart was planning to spend £30 million, or about $50 million, to reformulate its product line, adding that, "in the main, taste will be unaffected." Is that worth a third "wow"?

Clearly learning about this remarkable decision left *me* a little hyperactive! But when I calmed down and looked at it more closely, I discovered that Asda/Wal-Mart was far from the only corporation to respond to the Southampton Shocker in such a dramatic way. According to the Food and Drink Federation in England, several companies—whether British-based or British divisions of American corporations—had started offering their customers color- and additive-free processed foods. Is it just me, or do these companies sound positively eager to reassure British consumers that they've read the Southampton study and taken it to heart:

Coca-Cola Great Britain:

> "We are aware of the recent publication from the University of Southampton on selected artificial colours, and we will continue to follow the guidance of regulators on this issue."

And in fact, on May 27, 2008, the story broke that Coca-Cola was removing sodium benzoate from its products—but only in Great Britain.

Kraft Foods U.K.:

> "Kraft Foods UK has no products aimed at children that contain the ingredients highlighted in the FSA [Southampton] study. . . . [W]ith our recent Dairylea Lunchables reformulation in the UK, we reduced fat and salt, as well as removed artificial colours and flavours. Without compromising quality, taste and food safety, we will continue to see where we can make changes and still meet consumer expectations."

Mars U.K.:

> "We know that artificial colours are of concern to consumers, which is why, in 2006, Mars began a programme to remove them from our products. . . . [I]n November 2007, Starburst Chews became free from all artificial colours.˙. . . [I]n December 2007, Skittles were made free from all the artificial colours highlighted in a landmark study by Southampton University. . . . We have already removed four colours mentioned in the Southampton study from Peanut and Choco M&M's, and are in the process of removing the final one so they too will be free from these artificials during 2008."

Nestlé U.K.:

> "Nestlé UK does not manufacture children's products that con-
> tain any of the additives investigated by the FSA [Southampton]
> research . . . and from September 2007, the UK's favourite kids'
> chocolate brand—Milky Bar—is to be made with all natural in-
> gredients."

U.K. Cadbury Chocolate division:

> "We are committed to replacing all artificial colours in our sweets.
> We note the Southampton University findings, but we had begun
> this process already because we are continually listening to our
> customers."

I read over those quotes, and I just reeled. Why are companies that operate in Great Britain—including our very own U.S. companies, even
Kraft!—so eager to take out the artificial colors there and so completely
reluctant to do so here? Why are they willing to spend the money to re-
formulate their products there while refusing even to consider such a
changeover here?

Maybe the answer can be found in a BBC report on Asda/U.K. Wal-
Mart: "Explaining its decision to halt the use of artificial colours and
flavours, Asda said it was acting because 'mums and dads are becoming
more and more concerned about what's in the food they buy.'" An
Asda/U.K. Wal-Mart press release elaborates: "Reformulation was hard
work, but it was a labour of love." Well, why can't they perform that same
labor of love over here? What are we to them? And what are our kids?

So why do corporations in Great Britain—even U.S. corporations—
fall all over themselves trying to please British parents, while *our* concerns are simply brushed aside? Why do parents in Great Britain get to
shop with the confidence that their children's health is being protected,
while we U.S. moms and dads have to jump through hoops to protect our
kids? Why are U.S. corporations doing a better job of protecting kids
overseas than at home?

I can think of several reasons. One is that parents in Great Britain are simply more aware—and the corporations know it. The release of a single dramatic study, like the Southampton Shocker, really does motivate both public opinion and public policy in Britain, moving both corporations and governments to extraordinary measures. Here in the United States, we're so blinded by industry-funded research and industry-funded media that we don't even hear about the independent science being presented abroad. Or if we do, the news is soon drowned in a chorus of corporate voices talking about "junk science" and "tree huggers."

Then, too, the British government actually does regulate its corporations, rather than making a virtue of deregulation as we do here. As we've seen, our corporations literally send employees to go work for the FDA and other regulatory agencies, where they can write the rules that will govern their former—and often their future—employers. The British don't seem to have the same kind of revolving door that we Americans have or to give the same kind of power to corporate lobbyists.

Another factor has to be their health-care system. When people in Great Britain (and Europe and Australia) get sick, the government feels their pain—because the national health system has to pay for medical costs. That gives both taxpayers and government an incentive to keep health-care costs down, partly by demanding that corporations do everything possible to keep harmful products away from the public. Here in the United States, by contrast, our commercialized health-care system turns us each into little profit centers for the drug industry and the medical establishment, so there's no similar incentive to prevent health problems.

So for a number of reasons, corporations in Great Britain know that both citizens and their governments are going to respond to a study like the Southampton Shocker, one way or another. Maybe that's why they get on the stick and remove the offending ingredients *before* anyone has time to get upset that they haven't done so.

So again, I have to ask, *Why can't we have what they have overseas?* After all, we're not asking them to reinvent the wheel—they've already removed these ingredients from their products elsewhere. So why can't our children get the same protection? Why can't they serve up the same products to us?

As a proud American, it seems to me that our duty as moms and dads and concerned citizens is pretty clear. We have to get this information out there so that our government and our corporations listen to us, the way that governments and corporations in Europe, Australia, Great Britain, Japan, and other developed countries listen to *their* citizens.

Maybe Rumsfeld didn't want me to know all of this—after all I was only ten when it happened! But I know it now, and so do you. So pass it on! The health of our children depends on it.

Colin's New Deal

Every so often, you get those Mama moments that make all of the work worthwhile, and at the end of the summer of 2007, I got to have one of those moments. We were all sitting at the breakfast table, where Colin was enjoying his new dairy-free breakfast of a bagel, bacon, and fruit. Although he was still a conservative little boy, he now had a new bubbly personality that none of us had ever seen in him before and an occasional smile that cracked his face wide open in such a way that, as a friend of mine commented, "When that kid smiles, the whole world lights up!"

He was smiling now, laughing at some joke his sister had made, planning out his summer day with his younger brother. I felt such an incredible sense of relief just to see him so happy. I hadn't even consciously realized before that something had been wrong, but subconsciously, I know, I'd always been worried. Now I understood why.

We finished breakfast and Colin bubbled off, ready to enjoy his day. Then he circled back.

"You know what, Mommy?" he said to me. "My tummy and my head always used to hurt."

In that moment, I just wanted to wrap my arms around him, but I held back. Although Colin had graduated to bedtime hugs and nightly kisses, he was still one of those children who could be super-sensitive to the slightest touch. Instead I just said, as calmly as I could, "Oh, I didn't know that, Colin. Does it still hurt?"

"No," he said seriously. "It doesn't hurt anymore."

"Why not?"

"Because I don't drink milk."

"Oh," was all I could muster as I was flooded with Mama Guilt. How much pain had I inadvertently caused this child?

Colin went on. "I think by not having the milk or the yogurt, Mommy—I think that helped."

At that point, I could not resist, and I wrapped that boy in my arms. I told him how sorry I was that Mommy hadn't known all of this sooner. How sorry I was that I hadn't known how to help his tummy, his head, his ears, and their infections, his raw armpits that had embarrassed him at the swimming pool, his cough that had kept him awake at night. I told him I was so sorry that I had kept him on antibiotics that hurt his tummy, how sorry I was to have hurt him with food. And as I let go, I took his face in my hands and looked him in the eye.

"Here's the deal, Colin. I'm so glad you're telling me this. Because Mommy didn't know before, that she was giving you foods that made you hurt. But she knows this now, and you're helping Mommy learn. And from now on, whenever Mommy feeds you something that makes your head or tummy hurt, you tell me, okay?"

"Okay," said Colin, a bit *too* eagerly. I could see a glint of mischief coming into his eyes.

"But you have to be honest," I added quickly. "You *have* to tell the truth. You can't just say it about broccoli or carrots or food you don't like. You can't just say it because you don't feel like eating something. You have to really, really, really tell me the truth, Colin—you have to be honest and true, okay? That's our deal. Is that our deal?"

He thought about it a moment more. "Okay," he agreed. And then he did give me a hug. And then he bubbled off once more, ready to enjoy his day.

7

THE RING OF FIRE

By Christmas 2006, I'd started, slowly, to crawl out of the cave that I had buried myself in after so many traumatic discoveries so close together: That the politicians revered by my entire family had been so intricately involved in corporate deal-making at the FDA. That the food I'd fed my kids had, I now understood, endangered their health. That the system I'd believed in had, I now saw, been broken for quite a while. I sensed dimly that it was up to people like me—like all of us—to fix it. But I still wasn't sure we could.

Mindful of the lesson my little boy had taught me when he told me I needed a bigger team, I reached out. Around the time I sent my e-mail to Nell Newman, I also went to visit Father Rol, our parish priest. As I sat in his office, I found myself telling him about all the discoveries I had made and all the ways they had shaken me to my core.

Father Rol had been going through his own battle with a recent diagnosis of prostate cancer, so he could easily have turned away, unwilling to hear at such a time that his illness might have been triggered by the toxins in our food.

Instead, he believed me without hesitation, in a way that helped restore my faith in myself. He also told me something I've never forgotten.

"Robyn," he said, after listening to me pour out my doubts and frustrations and self-questioning and self-blame, "you're still trying to control what happens to you. You wish you could control how your parents and siblings react. You wish you could control what you find out and how it affects you.

"But when you are truly called to action, you have to let go of that control and really allow your faith to lead you. It is a fearful thing to fall into faith's hands." He smiled, entirely focused on me at that moment, despite his own pain. "What happens after that really isn't up to you."

I don't let too many people tell me things like that. But how could I not listen to Father Rol?

Later that week, I was out with my husband on our weekly date night. This was a tradition we'd started early in our marriage, when we realized that we needed to preserve a private, intimate time in the midst of our busy lives. When the kids came along, we were more grateful than ever that we'd made such a firm commitment to this kind of quiet night. We usually just went to our favorite little hole-in-the-wall bar where we shared nachos and beer.

That evening, as Jeff and I talked over our pile of nachos, it all just came pouring out. As I looked my kind husband in the eye, I told him how I felt that I had lost all trust in my belief system. I felt a betrayal as deep as I imagined it would feel if *he* had betrayed me, or lied to me, or turned out not to be the wonderful, honorable man I thought I'd married. I told him how sure I was that Nell Newman would never answer me, that no one would ever listen to me, that relations with my family would ever be restored. How hard it was to have learned such disturbing things, to hope for goals that might never be accomplished.

Yet despite my discouragement, I felt I could live with myself only if I tried to do everything that I could to help protect the health of our children—of all the children. I didn't know where this journey would lead me. But I knew I couldn't stop.

Jeff listened silently, the way he always did, until I had finished. Then he said, "Robyn, part of why people *will* listen to you is that you feel this way. You really believed that the system was supposed to work, and now you're finding out that it doesn't. I know that's hard—it's hard for me, too. But someone who was more cynical before, or more critical, might be dismissed. Your concern is so sincere—and I think people will get that."

Jeff's quiet certainty had a way of anchoring me, and for a moment, I couldn't speak. Then I said, "Are you really okay with all this? We're spending so much money to keep the Web site going. I'm spending so much time doing the research and reaching out to those who may never listen. So much of this falls on you and on the kids. And if I do somehow manage to get the word out, we don't know what will happen. What people will say about me . . . about us."

Jeff shook his head. "As long as we've got our health," he said, half-joking. Then he said, "You have to do what you believe in, Robyn. We both do. I don't think either of us would feel very good about walking away from this right now, no matter how it turns out."

The next week, I heard from Nell Newman's office, and, eventually, from Nell herself. Her support reassured me that I could, somehow, get the message out about the problems with our food supply and the need for things to be different.

Meanwhile, through a recommendation from Father Rol's assistant, I discovered a remarkable film, *The Future of Food*. I reached out to the producer, Deborah Koons Garcia, who saw immediately the connections between her work and mine. Deborah's film explored both the risks involved in genetic engineering and the political ties that had enabled it to progress so far. She also showed that Monsanto's harassment of farmers in the United States and Canada was part of a larger danger; that the increasing degree of corporate control over agriculture was posing a real threat to farmers, yes, but also to the environment and to our health.

When I discovered that Deborah was the widow of musician Jerry Garcia, I had to smile. I was so straight, I had never even owned a Grateful Dead album! Now, suddenly, I was a Southern-fried soccer mom joining forces with Jerry Garcia's widow, and in awe of her brilliant work.

But the real turning point came for me just after Christmas of that year. As I slowly began to share my story, I was told by several people that my "food crusade" reminded them of Erin Brockovich, so, as I had done to Nell Newman, I finally sent Erin an e-mail—cold. I don't even know whether I expected to hear back from her, though in my heart, I hoped to. With the Christmas season and all the emotional processing that the holidays engendered—I was still more or less estranged from my family—I was really more concerned with Jeff and the kids and the demands of daily life than anything else.

But that Christmas, I did hear from her, and it meant more than I can say. Knowing that someone I admired so much had taken the time to write to me, to tell me to hang in there—it somehow made all the other support I'd been getting come to life, as though finally I could let myself believe what I'd been hearing and what I knew in my heart to be true.

Inspired by Erin, I set about trying to reconnect with the allergy moms I'd met through my early work with FAAN. In February 2007, I joined them at a meeting to discuss what we could do to further raise awareness of food allergies, and I tried to share with them some of the discoveries I'd been making about genetic engineering and its relationship to allergies. I also tried to share what I'd learned about the FAAN medical board—the many ways that physicians and scientists were being subsidized by the food and biotech industries, and the influence that funding was having on the information we had access to.

No dice. Despite all the good work they were doing in their communities and with their families, these women just didn't seem ready to look at the big picture. Nor did they want to know that the doctors they revered were less than perfect—that those doctors might have forfeited their right to our trust.

I knew how these women felt. Less than a year ago, I had been just like them. But now, as Father Rol had said, I had stumbled upon a different truth. I couldn't go back.

Joining the Choir

All right. If the allergy moms didn't want to listen, then who *did* want to hear about the information I'd been discovering?

I realized that I'd been trying too hard to convince people who just weren't ready to listen to what I had to say. I was only one person, with limited time, resources, and energy. If I was going to get the message out, maybe I should start with a more sympathetic audience. Instead of being one lone voice singing in the wilderness, could I be part of a bigger choir?

Somehow these thoughts led me to Robert F. Kennedy, Jr. I knew that Kennedy had a kid with severe peanut allergies, so he would certainly grasp the urgency of the problem. And a friend of mine had heard a speech of his that month that was highly critical of Monsanto Corporation. Hmmm, if he already knew there was a problem with Monsanto . . .

I checked out Kennedy's book, *Crimes Against Nature,* and discovered how openly critical he was of what he saw as Monsanto's environmental misdeeds. I also learned that as a father of kids with food allergies and asthma, Kennedy had grown increasingly frustrated with FAAN's lack of progress in food allergy research, prompting him to start an alternate group, the Food Allergy Initiative (FAI).

Ironically, Drs. Hugh Sampson and A. Wesley Burks of the FAAN medical board had gone over to work with FAI as well. Like the allergy moms I had spoken with, Kennedy was probably unaware of their involvement with Monsanto, the Peanut Foundation, and other corporate groups. But maybe, unlike the allergy moms, Kennedy would be open to hearing about it.

I admit I was intimidated by the thought of Kennedy's political affiliations. The last thing I wanted was for the allergy issue to become partisan. Yet perhaps Kennedy, such a public Democrat, would be a good ally for me, the lifelong Republican soccer mom. Allergies and dangerous foods know no party lines and, ultimately, these issues would have to be exposed on a bipartisan stage.

All right then. Kennedy it was. Now, how should I reach out to him?

I remembered the presentations I used to make in my business school days, notebooks full of facts, figures, and analysis, set up to make an airtight argument with an enormous amount of information marshaled to prove my case. I decided to prepare a similar notebook on the genetic engineering issue, bringing in everything I'd learned. Just as I'd done when I was a grad student, I crammed for a deadline—in this case, my family's plan to visit my parents in March. I got the notebook ready, redrafted my cover letter at least twenty times, and sent the whole thing off. Then I left for Houston with Jeff and the kids.

The very day we returned, I got a phone call within an hour of walking in the door. To my shock and relief, it was Kennedy's chief of staff. She had me on speakerphone, so I shuttled all four kids into the backyard so that I could talk uninterrupted. All she kept saying was, "This is unbelievable."

A few days later, I was contacted by the producers from Kennedy's radio show, *Ring of Fire,* and invited to tape an episode. When I learned that they wanted to run it on Mother's Day weekend—the first anniversary of the official founding of AllergyKids—I couldn't help thinking how far I'd come.

The Kennedy connection proved to be a major turning point. Suddenly, people knew who I was—and, to my further shock, and, I guess, relief, they wanted to hear from me. In May 2007, I was invited to speak at a Chicago event for the organic industry where I had the pleasure of meeting a remarkable gentleman who represented Prince Charles.

Later that fall, Deborah Garcia recommended me to a producer on the *CBS Early Show* who was looking to do a segment on food. That appearance and an introduction from Prince Charles's representative led to an article about me in the *New York Times.* And that article, to my complete surprise, led to a flurry of interest from publishers, ultimately resulting in this book.

As I started to attract more media interest, people—often including the journalists who invited me on their shows—would ask me how it felt to have come this far. Had I expected to be in such demand? To receive so many invitations? To become "food's Erin Brockovich"?

I would try to explain that I didn't think of my work that way. I just wanted to get the message out. I mainly thought that we had to tell American moms what the European, Australian, Japanese, and Russian moms already knew: that we can make our food safe for our kids to eat and make laws to protect our children. My job, as I saw it, was to make sure this message was heard.

How could I do less? The safety of our children was at stake.

Fixing the FDA: Funding a Family-Friendly Solution

As I start to write this section in the summer of 2008, I once again think of the O'Jays' song "For the Love of Money," used as the theme of the show *The Apprentice: "Money, money, money, mo-ney!"* You can see that the FDA is in dire need of financial help just by reading the headlines. Beef recalls large enough to feed every American *two hamburgers!* Tomatoes with salmonella, spinach with *e. coli,* contaminated peanut butter!

And then there were the July 2008 articles in *The Economist* pointing out that in the previous twelve months, the price of food had risen by a whopping 66 percent and that the jump in June 2008 alone had been 11.3 percent!

That food has a hidden cost as well, because we also have to pay for all those appointments with pediatricians, specialists, and allergists when the food we buy makes our kids sick. And what about all those trips to the pharmacist to purchase more prescriptions for our children, who are quickly earning the title Generation Rx? (For more on *that* topic, check out the documentary film of that name.)

Even as we struggle to pay the grocery, doctor, and drugstore bills, we see our government allocating $600 billion of our tax dollars to the Pentagon's war efforts for the fiscal year of 2009 while granting only $2.4

billion to the FDA "to protect the health of the American public." That translates into the FDA receiving only *two days'* worth of military spending to protect consumers, regulate the food industry under the guidance of a "secretary of food," and investigate the safety of all food and drugs.

This whole situation gives new meaning to the phrase "penny-wise and pound-foolish," because underfunding the FDA is directly related to those doctor and pharmacy bills. The FDA itself stated in a November 2007 report that "American lives are at risk" as a result of the FDA's lack of resources. The agency says point-blank that at this level of funding, it "can no longer ensure the safety of the food supply."

Wait—*what?* It was bad enough when the FDA and Monsanto were passing the responsibility for testing new foods back and forth between them like some kind of toxic hot potato. Now the FDA is saying that it doesn't have the money to do *any* of its job? Even while Monsanto's profits continue to climb at an astronomical rate? When Monsanto announced its earnings in June 2008—the latest date available as of this writing—the company's shareholder dividends had jumped by 37 percent. That's no flash in the pan, either: according to an article called "Monsanto on the Menu" that ran in the June 2008 edition of *Business Week,* Monsanto's stock price rose by more than 1,200 percent between 2003 and 2008, while the FDA withers on the vine.

Now, why does this situation exist in the first place? Why aren't we raising a national outcry to fund the agency that's supposed to protect us and our children from toxins and other dangers in the food supply? Is our federal budget in such dire shape because of the resources being allocated to the Pentagon? Why do the food safety agencies of other countries warn parents away from, say, soy formula, while our own U.S. agencies fail to engage a public debate about such dangers? In Great Britain, the federal food safety agency actually funded the Southampton Shocker, the study that led to even U.S. corporations eliminating synthetic colors and sodium benzoate from their U.K. products. Why can't our own FDA take the lead in protecting us that way?

I have to believe that part of the problem is that unlike other countries, we have a privatized health-care system in which Big Pharma profits from how unhealthy we are, even as the food and biotech companies profit from what they sell us. In the current commercialized setup, no one has an incentive to keep us healthy: neither the companies that sell us the food we eat nor the corporations that make the drugs we buy. Whether it's my three-year-old with allergies or my father with heart problems, we're all seen as little profit centers.

In other countries, the health-care situation is quite different. Health-care systems are often paid for by tax dollars because they are the public responsibility of the government, not the profit centers of pharmaceutical corporations. As a result, both the government and the citizenry as a whole have a vested interest in making sure that everyone stays healthy. Is that why so many European countries have taken a stronger stand on food issues?

Meanwhile, in May 2008, our own Environmental Protection Agency literally lowered the value of a human life by nearly $1 million—from $7.8 million to $6.9 million, to be exact. That figure is used to assess corporate liability when a company's actions put a life at risk. By lowering the value of a human life, in other words, the EPA has reduced potential liabilities for U.S. corporations. Pretty convenient for capitalism, but not for our health and well-being. Are our lives really worth less today than they were a few years ago?

So here's one modest proposal. Given that food is largely responsible for making us sick and that in our commercialized health-care system pharmaceutical corporations are profiting off that illness, perhaps we should at least separate the "food" and "drug" components of our underfunded FDA and create a "Chinese wall" between the two agencies.

Certainly we should also increase the agency's funding, and maybe we should consider other options for delivering health care. But at the very least, we might consider having two separate agencies as other developed countries do: one whose entire mission is to supervise and regulate the food industry, and another with the goal of doing the same for the drug industry.

Is that so far-fetched? Not if you take a look around the world. It makes you wonder whose interests are being protected when here in the United States we have the two in bed together.

I also think that whoever is regulating food and drugs needs to focus more on children. In 1946, Harry Truman said, "A nation is only as healthy as its children." Well, Houston, we've got a problem! All too often, as we've seen, foods or food products that should be tested, aren't. But even when they are, they're usually tested on adults, particularly males, with no real analysis of how these results might translate when kids are involved.

I realize there are all sorts of ethical and practical problems in testing potentially toxic foods and drugs on children. But at the very least, their effect on children should be factored into the analysis of whether or not they're safe. As we saw with the StarLink scandal, this often isn't done—with potentially disastrous results for our kids. Maybe we should follow the lead of the New Zealand government and create a chief advisor for child and youth health.

In the same spirit, whoever tests food, drugs, and anything else we consume needs also to test ingredients in combination, not just singly. Recall Dr. David Ludwig's point from chapter 2: that he's less concerned about the effects of one single color or preservative than about the way everything interacts together. It kind of reminds me of high school chem class—you know, when they give you one vial of blue stuff and one vial of yellow stuff, and they're both just sitting there, and then you pour the two liquids into the same beaker, and suddenly they start to froth and smoke? It's not enough to know what each will do alone; we need to know how they behave in context. The Southampton Shocker was un- usual in that it tested children on a combination of two ingredients: tar- trazine (Yellow 5) *and* sodium benzoate. The study's designers knew that a child very rarely has occasion to ingest *just* a synthetic color or *just* a preservative; rather, a child who is gobbling up multicolored candies is probably taking in several colors and at least one preservative. We need to see more of that kind of thinking—and that kind of testing. You know, maybe a Sacramento Study or an Indianapolis Investigation. It might be a first, but wouldn't you be proud to see our studies heralded by moms in Europe?

And finally, since it all comes down to money, maybe it's time that we take a look at the U.S. Department of Agriculture's subsidy program and the billions of dollars being sent to farmers, executives, and others on the USDA payroll. Perhaps we should consider reallocating those taxpayer resources in a way that makes sense for the health of all of us.

Industry Stirs the Pot

I don't know about you, but when I think about the kind of tests that should be done—but aren't—my next question is *why?* Why aren't foods, additives, and preservatives tested in such a way that we get accurate, complete information about how they'll affect our children? And why, for that matter, are so many of the studies that *do* give us good information coming out of Great Britain, Italy, Australia, Russia—anywhere but our own United States?

When I began to answer this question for myself, I won't lie to you: I felt horribly discouraged. Because what I had to accept was that many of the U.S. scientists, physicians, and government officials who conduct and analyze food-safety tests were, to put it simply, working for private corporations.

Maybe they were doing so indirectly, as with all the Monsanto and Searle personnel spinning through that revolving door. Maybe they were doing so directly, as with the pediatric allergists who were inventing products for Monsanto or taking grants from the Peanut Foundation.

However the money flowed, though, I have to believe it made a difference. You can't tell me that a man or woman who's taking hundreds of thousands of dollars from a private corporation is going to feel fully able to come up with information that the corporation doesn't like. Maybe there are one or two saints out there, but the vast majority of the human race just isn't up to it. I know I wouldn't be! Either I'd open my big mouth once too often and get defunded, or I'd look at my kids' college funds and keep my mouth shut.

The problem extends beyond individual doctors and scientists to our major research institutions. Universities and research institutes depend on private funding, which appears to affect the way their professors and scientists think, act, and publish.

Look, for example, at the University of California's relationship with Monsanto. Together, the private corporation and the public university developed rBGH, the growth hormone used to make Monsanto's product Posilac, which farmers buy to boost milk production. (For more on rBGH, see chapter 4.) In order to avoid potential legal battles, Monsanto eventually paid the university a settlement of $100 million—*plus* it agreed to fork over fifteen cents for every dose of Posilac administered to every dairy cow. That means that as long as Posilac is sold and used, the University of California is receiving quite a hefty sum, year in, year out.

Now how is the University of California supposed to produce honest research on the dangers of genetic engineering and of rBGH in particular with that kind of financial interest in a genetically engineered product? And indeed, one of the university's biotechnologists and geneticists, Alan McHughen, is one of the nation's leading advocates of genetic engineering, having recently served on a panel at BIO 2008, a biotech industry conference. Author of the book *Pandora's Picnic Basket: The Potential and Hazards of Genetically Modified Foods,* Dr. McHughen has suggested that we put our trust in the FDA: "Most of us have a high degree of faith in our regulatory agencies. We can't argue with the record: No one has been made ill from eating genetically modified foods."

Well, that's one way of looking at it. Or we could look at the criticisms of the StarLink investigation (see chapter 5), the research suggesting that GM foods are allergenic (see chapter 3), the list of ailments related to GM soy discovered in the York laboratory study (see chapter 3), and the possibility that genetically modified foods, including rBGH, are indeed contributing to long-term health problems (see chapter 4).

Don't get me wrong: I'm not impugning Dr. McHughen's integrity. I'm only pointing out that given the recurring revenue stream from the university's royalty agreement with Monsanto, his institutional home has a vested interest in defending genetic engineering, an interest that might make it difficult for colleagues with different views to find funding, tenure, or institutional support.

I don't mean to point the finger at the University of California, either, because lots of universities are in the same boat—and often, they're in that boat with Monsanto. In 1985, for example, Cornell University did some research on rBGH for Monsanto, testing the product on dairy cows and sharing the findings with Monsanto to use in its FDA application. Cornell performed this service in exchange for a half-million-dollar grant, which entitled Monsanto to complete control of the university's research. According to an article in the January/February 1997 issue of *Mother Jones,* "computers in the university's dairy barn sent the raw data directly to Monsanto in St. Louis," so that "the company, rather than the university's principal research scientist, controlled and interpreted the data."

Now again, I'm not saying that Cornell *shouldn't* have taken the money. I'm not even saying they shouldn't have let Monsanto control the data—though my friends in the scientific community might think otherwise. I am saying that Cornell had a vested interest in discovering the data that Monsanto needed to make its case to the FDA, and that it continues, perhaps, to have a stake in supporting—or at least, not overly criticizing—the kinds of genetic engineering that it was once funded to study.

The problem is compounded by the fact that in order to get FDA approval for their products, private corporations *have* to fund research— that's the way the system works. They have to show the FDA that they've done the "due diligence" to ensure that the product they want to market will do what they promise and won't hurt anyone in the process. So they have to pay for research—and since they tend to have more money than anyone else, that makes them the best employer in town. Do *you* want to be the maverick scientist whom no industry will ever hire, perhaps no university either, because your very presence makes big funders a bit leery of getting involved with your institution?

Dr. Conflict of Interest—or Make That Interest(s)!

When I first learned of the financial ties between Big Pharma, Big Food, and the doctors whom we in the food allergy world had come to revere, I was overwhelmed by the seemingly endless list of financial ties. The doctors who were on the medical board of FAAN, for example, had multiple connections to both the food and the drug industries, having been funded by corporate research grants or involved in corporate research projects to an extent that I found shocking.

The first man I looked into was Hugh Sampson, MD. Dr. Sampson's work in the food allergy world has been extensive. One pediatric allergist in Los Angeles even referred to Dr. Sampson as "the pope of food allergies." Not only had Dr. Sampson been part of the StarLink corn investigation, but he had also conducted research for the FDA on additives like aspartame and bovine lactoferrin, a milk protein that is used as a binding agent in vaccines and processed foods.

But this same eminent scientist also had significant ties to the corporation responsible for creating and marketing genetically modified crops. Notably, Dr. Sampson was actually listed as a coinventor of one of Monsanto's patented and genetically engineered seeds. According to the U.S. Patent and Trademark Office, he had worked with Monsanto scientists to develop the kinds of products that, only five years earlier, he had warned might be the source of new types of allergens.

When I first discovered these corporate ties, I have to admit that it made me sad, as they seemed to highlight the flaws in our system: dedicated, talented scientists are so often employed by corporations who have a financial stake in the outcome of their research, while comparable funds don't seem to be available from independent sources. As a result, it's hard for the public to know how to view the scientific information we're given, since so much of the funding comes from companies with a built-in incentive to support research that will help their bottom line and profitability.

I was especially struck by how FAAN, the premier allergy nonprofit, appeared to have been affected by this system. Even though members of their medical board had pioneered inquiries into the links between genetic engineering and allergies, and into the potential cross-reactivity of peanuts and soy, the organization itself had remained silent on those issues. So had many of these same pioneers, at least in their public writings and statements. But if genetically modified crops were indeed creating new allergies—a possibility that Dr. Sampson himself had once highlighted—wasn't it their responsibility as physicians to keep speaking out?

Next, I looked into FAAN medical board member A. Wesley Burks, MD, one of the most trusted names in the world of pediatric allergy and immunology, renowned for the depth of the research he's conducted for the University of Arkansas and Duke University in the field of food hypersensitivity. For the last several years, according to ScienCentral News, Dr. Burks has been trying to develop a peanut allergy vaccine. Given how pervasive—and how deadly—the peanut allergy has become, Dr. Burks is truly pursuing the holy grail of the allergy community, and for this reason and others, is lauded by parents around the world.

Imagine my disappointment, then, when I discovered Dr. Burks also had corporate ties: in his case to Big Pharma *and* Big Food. According to an article in the March 13, 2003, *New England Journal of Medicine,* coauthored by Dr. Burks, "Dr. Burks has reported receiving consulting fees from Unilever, Wyeth, and Monsanto; receiving a grant and holding stock options and related patents with SEER (formerly Panacea); and receiving grants from the Peanut Board, the National Peanut Foundation, and Monsanto."

But these weren't Dr. Burks's only corporate ties. According to a June 2008 article in the *Journal of Allergy and Clinical Immunology,* Dr. Burks "has consulting arrangements with [pharmaceutical corporations] Acto-GeniX NV, Novartis, McNeil Nutritionals, and Mead Johnson; owns stock in [the biotech corporation] Allertein Therapeutics, LLC, [the pharmaceutical company] MastCell, Inc; is on the advisory board for Dannon Co. Probiotics [a nutraceutical company]; is on the speakers' bureau for EpiPen/Dey [a pharmaceutical manufacturer]; is on a data monitoring committee for Genentech [another pharmaceutical manufacturer]; is on an expert panel for Nutricia [a maker of medical foods and hypoallergenic infant formulas]; has received research support from the National Institutes of Health, Food Allergy and Anaphylaxis Network, Gerber [a baby food company], and Mead Johnson [a Bristol-Myers Squibb nutritional company that makes Enfamil, one of the most widely distributed infant formulas] . . ."

The corporate tie that leapt out at me from that list was the one with Dey Pharmaceuticals, which makes EpiPens, used to give emergency epinephrine injections to allergy and asthma victims suffering from anaphylactic shock. I wish I could give you the exact date that Dr. Burks began his relationship with Dey, but I can't. What I can tell you is that Dey Pharmaceuticals is an affiliate of Merck KGaA. And according to research from the American Academy of Allergy, Asthma and Immunology (AAAAI), Dr. Burks was part of that company's Speakers' Bureau.

Wow. Dey's public relations department must love seeing Dr. Burks appear in food allergy articles urging us to buy things like EpiPens. But how many of his patients and how many of his readers would have viewed this man's opinions the same way had he been wearing a baseball cap with the EpiPen logo, or Monsanto's or Dannon's or Gerber's?

These corporate ties raised another set of troubling questions: If the livelihood of doctors and scientists depends on the ongoing allergy epidemic, does the scientific community have any incentive to try to *prevent* this disease in our commercialized health-care system? Is that why only a handful of scientists is inclined to look at the root causes behind the allergy epidemic—people like Drs. Joel Fuhrman, Kenneth Bock, and David Ludwig, who point to a toxic environment and substandard nutrition as central factors in the epidemic's growth? Is it because so many doctors are funded by Big Pharma that so few doctors seem willing to consider non-medical approaches to allergies, such as the diet suggested by the Feingold Association? As I took a step back and examined what motivation most physicians and scientists might have to tell the truth, the whole truth, and nothing but the truth, I realized that, on the contrary, most of them had a far greater financial incentive to come up with answers that are amenable to their corporate funders.

I'm not saying that this is what happens in every case. I'm just recalling the two studies pointing out that when corporations funded research, that research tended to find corporate products safe, whereas when research was independently funded, it often came to the opposite conclusion. To me, this says that our system is broken: the way we fund research is not the best way to insure independent, reliable answers. I don't want to point the finger at any one doctor, because any one doctor may be perfectly ethical and honest. But overall, our system is broken, and we need to fix it.

Meanwhile, we can't continue to view these experts—despite their admitted knowledge and experience—as unbiased sources of information. Instead, we need to picture them wearing baseball caps with the name of their team—"Monsanto" or "BUY EPIPEN"—blazoned across the front! After all, when Kraft funded the development of FAAN's Web site, wouldn't you have taken the opinions on that page differently if you'd seen a Kraft logo there? When any research scientist who receives Monsanto funding chooses not to publicly address the potential relationship between GM foods and allergies, wouldn't you interpret his decision differently if he were wearing a Monsanto baseball cap?

Well, if these guys won't tell us where their money comes from—or if, like Dr. Burks, they bury the information in the fine print of scientific journals but don't post it on their groups' Web sites or in other easily accessible places—then we'll just have to find out this information for ourselves. Here's how:

1. *Whenever you read or hear an "expert opinion," consider the funding source.* Google the name of the doctor, organization, or medical institution and add one or more of the following terms: "disclosure," "speakers bureau," "grant," "consulting fee," or "funding." Chances are you'll hit a gold mine of information. I always do!

2. *Insist on full disclosure.* If the expert is not forthcoming in disclosing his or her funding, insist upon it. Take it up the chain

until you get it from someone at his or her organization. Then share the information: on your Web site, with your friends, in your blog, in e-mails. Get the word out.

3. *When considering these experts and their opinions, weigh the influence that patents, royalty fees, speaking arrangements, television appearances, and the like might have on their reputation and financial success.* Discuss this with your friends. How much money do these guys get from these corporate sponsorships? Start to picture them like those race car drivers who have their sponsorships and endorsements blazoned across their uniforms.

Once the experts know we're onto them, maybe they'll start disclosing this stuff for themselves. Better yet, maybe they'll start finding more independent and reliable funding sources.

Playing God in the Garden

If we're going to protect not only our children, but ourselves, I think all of us have to follow the lead of countries around the world and get serious about understanding and regulating genetic engineering. In France, for example, as of this writing, genetically modified seeds were not allowed to be planted in French soil, much less fed to French cows. Yet we are feeding these crops to our families, without ever having conducted human trials. Is that really the kind of health policy we want for our country?

In chapters 3, 4, and 5 of this book, you've had the opportunity to learn how genetic engineering works on different types of food, as well as to review how the GM process works in the first place. Now let's take a step back and look at the big picture: the moral, ethical, and practical dilemmas raised by genetic modification itself.

The phrase that to me best sums up the problem is Michael Pollan's evocative "playing God in the garden," which he first used in a 1998 *New York Times* article, presumably to express the depth of his concern about what might happen when humans could indeed "play God." What's disturbing to Pollan—and me—about genetic engineering is that not only are we manipulating the DNA of living organisms for our own purposes, but that we then take the process a step further and forcibly cross two living species that all the laws of nature have been designed to prevent from mating.

Sure, nature has mutated for centuries, creating new types of organisms. And of course, plants, animals, and species evolve. But to forcibly cross the DNA of two living organisms in a way that requires gene guns, bacteria, and viruses reminds me of taking someone against their will, creating a police state, or laying siege to a city. Of course, we can impose our will on others using guns and other types of violence, but what are the long-term consequences of such high-handed actions?

Above and beyond the ethical issues are the practical concerns. Since we've never been genetic engineers before, we don't know what happens when we start altering the basic genetic design of a plant—or, as is already happening, an animal, and perhaps someday, a human being. We don't know how the genetically engineered organisms will breed with the natural ones, and what might be the consequences of this "genetic roulette," to borrow the provocative title of author Jeffrey M. Smith.

Remember the studies from chapter 5 suggesting that GM crops produced skinny earthworms, weakened lacewings, and reduced populations of bees? Or the examples of the physicians who, in altering the genetic structures of viruses, inadvertently gave their patients new diseases?

I'm not saying we shouldn't explore this extraordinary technique, which may indeed fulfill its supporters' promises of defeating disease and overcoming starvation. But we need to know who's deciding which risks are okay and which are too dangerous. And we certainly need to know when corporate decisions affect not only the profitability of corporate product lines like herbicides and genetically modified seeds, but also the food we eat and the food we give our children.

There are also the political and economic concerns. So far, GM technology is pretty much the exclusive property of a handful of multinational corporations, chief among them, Monsanto. So even if we want *someone* to play God in the garden, we may not want to give *those* companies godlike power, using the patent and licensing process to create a global monopoly on virtually all the food that we eat.

Think of how powerful computers are and what an enormous difference computer technology has made to life on this planet. Then imagine what would have happened if the first company to make and distribute computers, IBM, had remained the *only* serious contender in the field. No Apple, no Mac, no Bill Gates, no Steve Jobs. That's the kind of monopoly that Monsanto has created for itself. And while the company that brought us DDT and Agent Orange may deserve praise for its forward-looking investment in biotechnology, I'm not sure it deserves to dominate global agriculture with its Roundup Ready soybeans designed to withstand increasing dosages (and sales!) of its Roundup herbicide.

In its rise to agricultural dominance, Monsanto has also racked up a pretty impressive record of corporate misdeeds. Here are just a few of its actions in recent years:

- In August 1999, Britain's Advertising Standards Authority charged the company with misleading the public about its genetically modified food and crops.
- In August 2000, a Philadelphia jury ordered the company to pay $90 million in damages to the state of Pennsylvania to help pay for selling defective and toxic PCBs that left the highly toxic chemical by-product that contaminated a government building.
- In February 2002, an Alabama jury found that Monsanto had engaged in "outrageous" behavior by dumping PCBs into the environment and then attempting to cover up its actions.

A quick Google search reveals an even longer list, but I'll jump to one of the more recent and more disturbing:

> • In December 2007, the company was brought up on charges in South Africa based on claims that, once again, Monsanto had misrepresented its genetically modified products, which had led to various types of false advertising.

Of course, the defenders of genetic engineering make some pretty good points, too. You've probably heard their responses; you may even have come up with some of them yourself. So let's look at the arguments *for* genetic engineering and take them on, one by one. Then you can make up your own mind—or start asking new questions of your own.

> 1. *People who oppose genetic engineering romanticize nature. But not everything natural is good. Nature can be harmful or beneficial to humans—just like science.* I personally love this argument because, having grown up in Houston, I don't think I ever *did* romanticize nature! I'm all for science making our lives easier, and I believe that technology and innovation will help us develop new solutions to our problems in ways that we might never have imagined.
>
> But nature has one advantage over science that I know of—it has its own sense of limits and balance. Changes in nature take time, and with our human ingenuity—and science—we often have a certain amount of time to respond to them.
>
> Changes made by humans, however, often happen in a very sweeping, overwhelming, and rapid way, and by the time we've figured out what their real consequences are, it may be too late to go back. By all means, let's explore the potential benefits of genetic engineering—but let's do so carefully and with a sense of humility. Let's invite many voices into the discussion and not allow our debate to be determined by the will of a single corporation presenting a few industry-funded studies. Above all, let's not rush ge-

netically engineered crops into production and into the fields before we have any real idea of how they'll affect our environment,
our health—or our children.

A global discussion might be a great place to start. Interestingly,
the Vatican had this to say about genetic engineering in a February 2005 report: "available scientific data are contradictory or
quantitatively scarce. It may then be appropriate to base evalua-
tions on the precautionary principle." The precautionary principle dictates that new technology or products shouldn't be
introduced into general circulation until we have some solid idea
of what their effects might be.

2. *Genetic engineering isn't really that different from the kinds
of breeding that farmers have been doing for hundreds of thousands of years. Many of the plants and animals we rely on now
are the result of generations of careful breeding. Genetic engineering just allows the process to go a little faster.*

Again, good point—but maybe incomplete. Sure, there's a way
that genetic engineering resembles the long, slow process that
gave us that plump, succulent ear of corn, rather than the tough,
gnarled cob that farmers grew five hundred years ago. But to say
that conventional breeding resembles genetic engineering is like
saying that a house cat resembles a tiger. Yes, there are similari-
ties—but the comparison leaves out some very important distinc-
tions.

As we saw in chapter 5, conventional breeding has its own
built-in limits. Nature won't allow DNA to mix if it comes from
species that are too far apart. Nor does nature create new types of
DNA "from scratch." Maybe from our human point of view, there
are shortcomings to the ways that nature works, but there are also
natural limits to how wrong things can go.

What's frightening about genetic engineering is that we're taking down barriers without knowing what possible dangers that will
unleash, much as if we mistook a tiger for a house cat and began
stroking its back. The tiger *might* purr and rub its head against our

leg—but if it decides to scratch, it's going to cause far more harm than that house cat ever could. Before we rush over to pet its lovely fur and invite it into our kids' bedrooms, let's learn a little bit more about what that tiger is capable of.

3. *The world needs food, especially the developing world. Genetically modified crops offer greater and more reliable yields. Even here in the United States, other than financing terms, there's a good reason that farmers have turned to GM crops—they make it possible for farmers to guarantee higher yields, safeguarding their livelihoods and preserving our farm community.*

Well, who could argue with this one? If there's even a small chance that genetically modified crops could make even a small dent in the global problems of hunger and malnutrition, how can we waste our time talking about skinny earthworms or even allergic reactions? Why aren't we embracing this promise with all the enthusiasm that it deserves?

I must admit, if GM crops really did offer the promise of ending world hunger, I'd be hard-pressed to malign them. While the Mama Bear in me would be insisting that Colin and Tory and Lexy and John mean more to me than some abstract family in India or Africa, the world citizen in me might be willing to take the risk.

However, the defenders of GM crops (who, if you look closely, tend to own either shares or patents in the companies that *make* these crops) are overstating their case in a number of ways. First of all, genetically modified crops *don't* necessarily produce higher yields. Remember those Texas farmers in chapter 5 who sued Monsanto because their cotton crops *didn't* resist insects as advertised? Well, they're not the only ones who noticed that GM crops aren't necessarily all they're cracked up to be.

According to the U.S. Department of Agriculture—hardly an anti-industry or antitechnology organization!—"currently available GE crops do not increase the yield potential of a hybrid variety. In fact, yield may even decrease if the varieties used to carry the herbicide-tolerant or insect-resistant genes are not the highest yielding cultivars."

In other words, engineering crops that can withstand weed-killer or bugs may make life easier for farmers. But they don't necessarily produce more crops, despite what the industry-funded research might claim. (And, as the farmers found in Texas, GM crops don't even always withstand what they've been bred to withstand!)

Furthermore, a 2004 report from the U.N. Food and Agriculture Organization on agricultural biotechnology acknowledges that genetically engineered crops can have *reduced* yields. *That* can't be good for the developing world.

Not convinced yet? Wait, there's more! A 2007 study by Kansas State University agronomist Dr. Barney Gordon suggests that Roundup Ready soy continues to suffer from what is colorfully known in agricultural circles as a "yield drag." Apparently Roundup Ready soy yielded 9 percent *less* than a close conventional relative. And according to a 2003 report published in *Science,* "in the United States and Argentina, the world's largest growers of genetically engineered soy, the average yield effects [of GM crops] are negligible and in some cases even slightly negative."

"Yield may even decrease . . ."

"Yield drag . . ."

"[A]verage yield effects are . . . in some cases even slightly negative . . ."

Doesn't sound like these genetically engineered crops are going to be ending world hunger anytime soon. Sure, these promises of greater outputs in the fields help to drive up the stock price of companies like Monsanto, but promises don't feed the hungry children in Africa.

Additionally, GM crops create problems of their own—problems that are often costly and sometimes environmentally dangerous to solve. Those skinny earthworms and weakened lacewings aren't just the poster creatures for some wild-eyed ecologist: they're a very real part of our agricultural process. If GM technology inadvertently kills these helpful organisms, we're going to need more technology to compensate. And what if that new technology creates still more problems, in an ever-growing vicious cycle that genuinely threatens our ability to produce food?

To some extent, you can see this kind of problem beginning with Monsanto's Roundup Ready soybeans. Genetically engineered to withstand spraying with Monsanto's herbicide Roundup, the beans engendered a whole other set of ecological problems. Because the weeds were being sprayed instead of removed in other ways, they developed their own resistance to the herbicide, creating the so-called "superweeds."

To kill superweeds, you need a super-herbicide—such as 2,4,5-T, conveniently also made by Monsanto. But do we really want all those chemicals being sprayed over our fields? And what if those superweeds come back to haunt us, choking those brave new crops that were meant to end world hunger?

Here's another concern: how does the spraying of all of these nitrogen-based chemicals affect the environment? The USDA has just waived pesticide reporting requirements for corporations like Monsanto, a procedure that has been in place since the early 1990s so that farmers and consumers would know the levels of chemicals being applied to food crops. You have to wonder what the long-term consequences of this "don't ask, don't tell" policy will be. And let's not forget that, according to the May 2008 *Vanity Fair* article, "Harvest of Fear," the USDA has its own share of former Monsanto employees in house.

Finally, as we've seen, the net effect of GM crops is to make farmers far more dependent on Monsanto. Just for the sake of having a more interesting sentence, I'd love to add a few more corporate names to that list, but I really can't: it's literally Monsanto that owns the patent on genetically modified seeds (as well as on the herbicides Roundup and 2,4,5-T).

So when farmers grow genetically modified soy, corn, cotton, and canola, they have to buy their seeds from Monsanto. And then, thanks to the patent system, they have to *keep* buying them. As we saw in chapter 4, Monsanto insists that farmers who have GM crops on their property for any reason—whether the farmers planted them or not—must pay for the privilege. Can you imagine if every time that you logged on to your computer you had to pay a licensing fee to Microsoft? In their most recent earnings announcement, Monsanto just highlighted that the price of corn seed is expected to go up 20 percent. I guess that's what comes of having a global monopoly on the food supply. It's great for the shareholders—but what about the rest of us?

In order to ensure the ongoing revenue stream that results from all of these repeat customers, Monsanto wants farmers to destroy seed from their crops every season so that they have to return to Monsanto for new supplies. Now that's asking a lot of a cash-crunched farmer—to destroy perfectly good seeds and then have to pay out for more.

Another cost to farmers is what seed companies term a "technology fee," charged on top of the already high price, supposedly to pay the company for the cost of having developed its patented technology. Including the fees, GM seeds typically cost farmers 24 to 40 percent more than non-GM seeds. For GM maize, costs run anywhere from 30 percent to 90 percent higher. All this to plant crops from which the farmer can't even save any seed.

In 2001, Dr. Charles Benbrook presented results of analysis of the economics of Bt maize (corn engineered with the insecticidal protein as discussed in chapter 5). He found that over three years, U.S. farmers paid large price premiums for GM seeds and ended with a net loss of $92 million or $1.31 per acre. Benbrook also found that the "planting of 550 million acres of GE corn, soybeans, and cotton in the United States since 1996 has increased pesticide use by about 50 million pounds." As we've seen, the "herbicide-tolerant" crops require far more use of special herbicides than normal plants and, indeed, have been specially developed to keep farmers buying herbicides from Monsanto. Is that why the USDA and the former Monsanto employees now within that agency agreed to waive the reporting requirements for pesticides?

I don't know about you, but allowing one single giant corporation that kind of worldwide power over the planet's food just plain makes me nervous. There may be some version of genetic engineering that really does improve crop yields while also preserving some kind of autonomy for the countries and communities that employ it. As of this writing, though, if you want to "go GM," you have to go Monsanto. Call me crazy, but giving one U.S.-based corporation virtually total power over all the food in the world does not seem like the right way to end world hunger.

There *has* to be a better way. Maybe allowing some market competition and exposing these government ties are a good place to start.

Throwing Caution to the Wind

Whenever I bring up the question of genetic engineering, someone says, sooner or later, "But that was banned in Europe—and then they changed their minds. If genetic engineering is okay with the Europeans, who are so much more careful about that stuff than we are, then it's probably safe, right?"

Well, no. That's not exactly what happened in Europe, a story that I actually find rather inspiring. So let me fill you in on the story of Europe and GM and you can decide for yourself.

Back in 1995, as genetically modified foods began flooding Great Britain and European markets, an acclaimed biologist named Arpad Pusztai was awarded a research grant to create a model for testing GM foods.

Dr. Pusztai was a widely respected scientist. He had published nearly three hundred scientific articles and twelve books, and was considered one of the world's leading scientists in experimental biology.

His colleagues were also widely respected, including scientists at the Rowett Research Institute in Scotland, the Scottish Crop Research Institute, and the University of Durham School of Biology. This consortium had been selected over twenty-seven other contenders to establish a standard that could be used in Britain and that would probably be adopted throughout the European Union. Its work would be the first research ever to be published evaluating the safety of GM foods, in this particular case, of potatoes.

The new protein that had been inserted into the potatoes' DNA enabled the spuds to produce their own insecticide—a natural insecticidal protein that was supposed to be safe for human consumption. By the time Pusztai and his colleagues received their grant, GM potatoes were already being consumed in the United States. If the research went the way everyone expected, the door would be opened for their introduction into Britain and Europe.

Given the widespread consumption of those potatoes, everybody involved in the research, Pusztai included, expected the scientists to conclude that feeding rats GM potatoes produced the same results as feeding them non-GM potatoes. But that wasn't what happened. Instead, to his astonishment, Pusztai discovered that genetically modified potatoes not only differed in nutritional content but in their effect on the animals in their study. After only a ten-day feeding study, animals fed the GM potatoes suffered damage to their immune systems, organs, and tissues, as well as other serious health problems.

Disturbed by this surprising outcome, Pusztai began compiling his findings for publication. While doing so, he was approached by producers for a British television show, *World in Action,* who were eager to break the story.

Now, scientists live by a strict code of ethics. They're not supposed to divulge their findings until their research has been published. That protocol is intended to safeguard the integrity of the research process. The scientist can't just talk about what he or she has done, possibly distorting or exaggerating it. Rather, the research must be vetted by the editors of the journal that publishes it and approved by the scientists' peers. It must also be available in its entirety for other scientists to criticize. "Just talking" about unpublished research gives the scientist a kind of unfair advantage, a way of getting his or her ideas out into the world without other scientists being able to evaluate or criticize them.

Pusztai wasn't some young, ambitious scientist, ready to break with

the code of ethics to make a media name for himself. He was a respected elder statesman in the scientific community, someone who had
nothing to gain and everything to lose by violating his profession's protocol.

Yet Pusztai decided that the safety concerns associated with GM potatoes were so great that he had to take a stand. Courageously, he broke
with his scientific code of ethics and agreed to appear on British television highlighting key aspects of his study.

Monsanto—the corporation responsible for those GM potatoes—had
already begun an all-out PR campaign, including full-page ads in British
newspapers touting the benefits of GM technology. So, in addition, by
speaking out, Pusztai was responding to an issue that was even then in
the process of being decided in British public opinion.

On August 10, 1998, Pusztai appeared on British television to share
the dangers he had discovered in GM technology. Speaking of the dangers of genetically modified crops, he said, "We are assured that: 'This is
absolutely safe. We can eat it all the time. We must eat it all the time.
There is no conceivable harm which can come to us.' But as a scientist
looking at it, actively working on the field, I find it very very unfair to use
our fellow citizens as guinea pigs. We have to find the guinea pigs in the
laboratory."

The press went wild. But within two days of publicizing his discoveries on British television, Pusztai was suspended from the institute where
he'd worked for more than thirty-five years and vilified by the same
British government that had funded his research. He was also placed
under a gag order that prevented him from discussing his findings any
further.

If Pusztai's story had ended there, Europe's relationship to genetic engineering might have been very different. But fortunately for European
consumers, the story had a second chapter.

The Genie Leaves the Bottle

Despite the gag order on Pusztai himself, the scientist's television appearance had let the genie out of the bottle. News of the dangers Pusztai had discovered created a groundswell of anti-GM sentiment in Great Britain.

Over time, other scientists rallied to Pusztai's defense. Former president of the British Society for Allergy and Environmental Nutritional Medicine Ronald Finn said, "Dr. Pusztai's results at the very least raise the suspicion that genetically modified potatoes may damage the immune system. You can imagine a doomsday scenario. If the immune system of the population was weakened, then the mortality would be increased many, many times."

The Pusztai affair was barely mentioned in the U.S. press. But it made headlines in Britain and rocked public opinion throughout Europe as well. As with the Southampton Shocker, European public response moved corporations—even U.S.-based ones—to take actions that consumers wanted, even before the government demanded it. As a result, in April 1999, according to author Jeffrey Smith, "the British food industry bowed to consumer pressure. Unilever, England's biggest food manufacturer, announced that it would remove GM ingredients from its products sold in Europe. Nestlé made its announcement the next day, as did the major supermarket chains including . . . Safeway, (Wal-Mart's UK division) Asda . . . and McDonald's and Burger King also committed to remove GM soy and corn from their ingredients in European stores."

The European Union went on to pass a law requiring the labeling of foods containing ingredients with more than 1 percent GM content. The British Medical Association joined the chorus, calling for a moratorium on planting GM crops commercially and warning that "such food and crops might have a cumulative and irreversible effect on the environment and the food chain." In 2003, the European Parliament took regulation a step further and voted to lower the labeling threshold to 0.9

percent. And in October of 2007, Russian president Vladimir Putin signed a law doing the same in Russia.

Europeans were also concerned about Monsanto's control of GM technology. As a result, Monsanto found itself locked in a nine-year legal battle as it fought the European Patent and Trademark Office for the monopoly rights to European Patent no. 301,749, to "all forms of genetically engineered soybean varieties and seeds, regardless of the genes used." Europeans were unwilling to allow a single corporation to control such powerful technology—though Monsanto did eventually win that battle.

In an apparent effort to win support and to counter the small number of truly independent research efforts, Monsanto and the biotech industry funded their own research. For example, Monsanto finances the Kenya Agriculture Research Institute studies of Dr. Florence Wambugu, whose studies claim that GM crops could raise crop yields by four to ten tons per hectare. However, Dr. Wambugu's critics maintain that the descriptions of her GM crop yields were exaggerated.

In June 2003, it seemed that the supporters of GM technology had won a decisive victory when U.K. prime minister Tony Blair fired Michael Meacher, his minister for the environment, a known critic of genetic engineering. But opposition to genetic engineering continued. For example, in January 2004, the Soil Association spoke out. This venerable British group was respected around the world as a major authority on agricultural issues. The organization warned against genetic engineering, declaring, "The only human GM trial so far found that GM DNA transferred to bacteria in the human gut, while animal trials have seen a doubling of death rates among chickens fed GM feed and the development of gut lesions in rats eating GM potatoes and tomatoes."

As we saw in chapter 5, the transfer of genetically modified DNA to bacteria in the human gut is a huge concern. In theory, genetically modified DNA is supposed to pass through our digestive system and be eliminated. No one knows the potential consequences of altering the DNA of our intestinal bacteria. Are Monsanto and the FDA each going to keep insisting that it's the other one's job to ensure food safety?

News articles continued to fan the flames in 2003 and 2004 by reporting that Britain's mad-cow scare might well have been the result of feeding cattle genetically modified feed.

So, if we are to step back from this political and scientific muddle, what is going on in Europe today? Obviously, Europe is still worried about the potential dangers of these crops, including the cross-contamination of non-GM plants, damage to livestock from GM feed, increased pesticide use on pesticide-resistant crops, technology fees charged to farmers, environmental damages, and the lack of human trials.

Now it's true that the EU has bowed to U.S. pressure and allowed the planting of GM crops. But public opinion—and farm opinion—continues to oppose genetic engineering. If you listen to the biotech industry, you'll hear that 2007 saw a 77 percent increase in GM corn cultivation in Europe. But take a step back and you'll realize GM corn can be found on only 2 percent of the total European land allotted to growing corn. Despite government acquiescence, farmers and consumers stand firm.

And what about Arpad Pusztai? What happened to genetic engineering's first whistle-blower?

Well, in October 1999, his research was finally published in *The Lancet,* Britain's most prestigious medical journal. And the eminent scientist is still trying to warn us about the dangers of genetic engineering:

> The situation is like the tobacco industry. They knew about it but they suppressed information. They created misleading evidence that showed that the problem wasn't so serious. And all the time they knew how bad it was. Tobacco is bad enough. But genetic modification, if it is going to be problematic, if it is going to cause us real health problems, then tobacco will be nothing in comparison with this. The size of genetic modification and problems it may cause us are tremendous. People should be made accountable for the crimes they committed.

So here's my question. If Europeans are still hesitant to put GM seeds in their soil or feed GM crops to their cows, and if they continue to insist on labeling GM ingredients at levels of less than 1 percent, then what in the world are we doing here in the United States feeding unlabeled genetically engineered foods to *our* children?

Patently Absurd: The New Trend of Patenting Genes

Okay, so here's where the story gets *really* weird. Monsanto isn't just patenting the seeds used to grow genetically modified corn, soy, and other crops. It's also trying to patent pigs.

That's right. Pigs. Not just seeds. Not just genes. Not just methods of breeding. But actual pigs.

The patent applications were discovered by Greenpeace researcher Christoph Then, who found that they had been published in February 2005 at the World Intellectual Property Organization (WIPO) in Geneva.

"If these patents are granted," Then says, "Monsanto can legally prevent breeders and farmers from breeding pigs whose characteristics are described in the patent claims, or force them to pay royalties. It's a first step toward the same kind of corporate control of an animal line that Monsanto is aggressively pursuing with various grain and vegetable lines."

Are you shocked? The researcher was, too. "I couldn't believe this," he says. "I've been reviewing patents for ten years and I had to read this three times. Monsanto isn't just seeking a patent for the method, they are seeking a patent on the actual pigs which are bred from this method. It's an astoundingly broad and dangerous claim."

So, how is this going to work? If you're a farmer who buys a pig bred in the Monsanto way, do you have to pay royalties on the pig for life? Do you have to pay a licensing fee for every pig that descends from the Monsanto "original"? Will Monsanto monitor this, the way they currently monitor farmers who inadvertently grow Monsanto GM crops when some seed accidentally blows onto their land? (See chapter 4 for more details on *that* story.)

What if you have a pig that simply *resembles* the Monsanto pig? Does Monsanto get paid for that pig, too, since they can claim you bred your pig to resemble theirs, just as a computer manufacturer who found you replicating a patented computer could claim that you were illegally copying their machine?

If it's scary patenting a pig, what do you think about the notion of patenting a *human* gene? Well, that, too, has already happened.

In 1994, the *New York Times* reported on a dispute between the U.S. government and a Utah company, Myriad Genetics, Inc., over the right to patent BRCA1, a gene that puts women at risk for breast cancer.

The gene was discovered by a team of scientists that included people from the National Institutes of Health, the University of Utah, and Myriad Genetics, Inc. Now let's be very clear: this isn't a genetically engineered lab creation we're talking about. This is an actual, natural gene, one that lurks inside the bodies of some 600,000 U.S. women, putting them at risk for breast cancer. Being able to identify this gene means that we can test people for it, enabling hundreds of thousands of women to take more aggressive cancer-prevention steps than they otherwise might. Understanding the gene might also lead to treatments that could stop some kinds of cancer in its tracks.

This is all a good thing, right? As a woman who's been drinking IGF-1-laden milk and eating rBGH yogurt for way more years than I wish I had, I think it's a *very* good thing.

But then the university and the private company went on to patent the gene. Literally, they wanted to own the rights to a human gene.

This boggles my mind. How can anyone own the rights to a piece of genetic material that appears inside the bodies of 600,000 women?

It's pretty clear why the university and the company wanted the patent. Ownership of the gene gave them a financial piece of any diagnostic test done to identify it and any treatment developed on the basis of it. But is that right? I mean, yes, they should be rewarded for their work and investment—but owning a gene that may be part of my body? Or yours?

The dispute arose because the NIH and its scientists were left off the patent, which didn't sit right with Oregon senator Ron Wyden. According to the *Times* article, "Mr. Wyden had put pressure on the institutes to insure that BRCA1 would be used for the public good and fairly priced, because the Government had a role in the discovery and the research had been partly financed by taxpayers."

Another critic of the action was Fran Visco, president of the National Breast Cancer Coalition. The *Times* quotes her as saying, "Women gave their blood for this research. I know many of these women, and they didn't give blood so some company could make millions of dollars."

In 2004, the European Patent Office revoked Myriad Genetics' patent, terminating its exclusive rights to perform diagnostic tests for BRCA1. But here in the United States, the patent still stands. So if your sister, your daughter, or your mom is carrying the breast-cancer gene in her body, then Myriad Genetics owns that piece of her anatomy. And if you wanted to develop a test to determine the role that rBGH plays in the development of breast cancer, as evidenced by the increase in the hormone IGF-1 and its impact on tumor growth, you could only do so if you were granted permission by Myriad Genetics to use this gene in your studies, since they now own the patent.

So if Myriad Genetics were to decide that pursuing research that links rBGH to breast cancer is not in their best interest (say, they would rather develop a blockbuster drug to treat the disease than have people stop drinking carcinogenic milk), they could refuse to grant you a license to their patented breast-cancer gene, effectively curtailing your research. And should you be bold enough to conduct the research *without* their license, they could sue you. What have we come to?

Mama Steps

So now that we've seen how dangerous our food has become, the next question is, *What do we do about it?*

I hope I've made it clear by now that first and foremost I am a mom who happened to have a background in research and finance. I don't think of myself as an activist any more than I think of myself as a cook. Instead, I see myself as a mother with four kids who's doing everything she can to make the world better for them.

In my more optimistic moments, I hope I'm being a good role model for my kids. I hope I'm teaching them—my girls as well as my boys—that we all have a responsibility to one another. That when something is wrong, you figure out what the problem is and then you work on solving it by doing your homework and building a team. That when something is unfair, you figure out how to make it fair. That when people are being hurt—whether members of your own family or people you've only heard about—if you can do something to help them, you do.

Somehow, this journey I've taken—this journey that was thrust on me—has given me a new sense of responsibility. Simply put, I now believe that *we* are responsible for our health and the health of our children. Not the president, not Congress, not the Monsanto Corporation, not the FDA. *We* are, mothers and fathers, citizens and consumers, all of us who are capable of learning what the problem is and doing something about it—we're responsible to do it. You know that quote "All that's needed for evil to triumph is for good people to do nothing"? Well, if I've learned nothing else these past two years, I guess I've learned that. But since I'm a "make lemonade" kind of person, let's turn it around: All that is needed for good to triumph is for good people to do *one* thing.

So think of the good that you have already done in learning all of this, and of all the ways that you can now protect the health of your family and friends. And if you want a few more suggestions, then read on. There are lots of ways to take action. Here are some that may work for you:

Find Out More

The first step is just learning what's going on and talking about it. I am grateful that you have taken the time to read this book, for starters. Now talk about what you've learned with your husband, your wife, your sister, your neighbor, your best friend, the woman behind you in the grocery line. Share your knowledge with those who might not have the time, energy, or resources to have learned what you now know. Talk about how Kraft uses chemicals in our American boxes of mac 'n' cheese even though they've removed those same chemicals from their boxes in England. Tell people that Safeway and Wal-Mart have labeled GM ingredients in Europe but not here. You will have so much fun teaching people about this, as it's such eye-popping information!

You don't have to stop with the material in this book, either. Check out some of the other books I recommend in the Resources section, or go to one of the Web sites I suggest. Get onto Google or some other search engine, and put in the terms that you want to find out more about. Subscribe to some newsletters, mix it up!

Listen to what activists like Jeffrey Smith at www.SeedsofDeception .com have to say, and balance it with the *New England Journal of Medicine*'s newsletter. Choose a few Web sites from overseas to visit. Two of my favorites are www.FoodNavigator.com and www.TakePart.com and their film, *Food, Inc.* Pick out a favorite blogger or two. Not only do you get some pretty wild information, but it can also be pretty entertaining. One of my favorites is the Renegade Lunch Lady, Chef Ann Cooper, at www.lunchlessons.org. Her sense of humor is essential when hearing some of this appalling information.

Pair Up with Some "Food Buddies"

It's so much easier to do *anything* when you don't feel isolated! So find a friend! If you're trying to make some positive changes in your kitchen, maybe like the ones I suggest in chapter 8, you may run into resistance from your husband, kids, or even your family of origin. For almost two years, my sons wouldn't eat carrots if you paid them five dollars a stick, and you don't want to know what my siblings said about my new regime! Luckily for me, Jeff was always super-supportive, but I look back and realize how much easier the process would have been if I'd known two or three other women who were going through it with me.

So learn from my mistakes: find some companions along your journey. You'll be doing yourself a favor and them as well. Even if it's only two of you in the beginning, you *will* create a buzz, as this taps into every Mama Bear instinct out there. And when people overhear you on the playground, maybe they'll want to learn more, too.

Get Involved at Your Kid's School or Preschool

You can certainly do what I did and just make your kids' lunches yourself. But if that's not an option, either because of your own schedule or because of your child's preferences, you have a built-in motivation to lobby for some healthy, kid-friendly choices in schools. Lots of schools have snack-food machines or soda machines, too, which might also be an issue that concerns you.

If you do want to push your school to offer some better options, here are some tips for how to move things forward:

FIND SOME ALLIES. You'll have more impact if you're not the only one raising the issue. You can divide up the work, too. And with others on your team, you'll just plain have more fun. Talk to other moms when you drop off or pick up your kids, or when you arrange play dates, or when you show up at parent-teacher night or attend some other school event. See who else would like to make some small but powerful changes.

DO YOUR HOMEWORK. Have other schools in your area offered healthier choices in the lunchroom or in their vending machines? What about adding a salad bar in the cafeteria? What kinds of food would be both kid-friendly and healthy? Is there a local nutritionist or scientist who can help you figure out some specifics? You'll make a stronger case if you've done some of this background work—and you'll feel more empowered and sure of yourself, too.

SET UP A MEETING. Find out who's got the decision-making power and set up a meeting. If you can manage it, don't go alone—there's not just safety and strength in numbers, but confidence, too! Let the person who makes the appointment know that there will be at least three of you.

GET THE MEDIA INVOLVED! You have to remember that journalists these days are moms and dads just like me and you. They've got kids with ADHD, kids with allergies, sisters with breast cancer, and dads who have battled prostate cancer. They want to know what you know, but in the busyness of their careers, they might not have found the time to learn it. You will be *amazed* at how responsive they are. Let them know about your meetings, invite them to join your groups, and remember that they are always looking for new things to write about. And the added publicity might just put a little pressure on the school.

PLAN THE MEETING. Ideally, you'll each say something, making three separate, powerful points. That's usually all you'll have time for before letting the person you're meeting with respond. Figure out the three most important ideas you want to share and divide them up among yourselves. Rehearse your presentations for one another—about two minutes each is a good amount of time—and give one another feedback on how to strengthen your approach. If someone in the group is very shy, she doesn't have to speak—she can just come along for moral support. She may surprise herself—and you—by discovering that she has something to say after all.

HAVE A CLEAR, DOABLE REQUEST. Meetings work best when they're based around a clear action. If you go in with a specific request, both you and the person you're meeting with will have a better idea of where the meeting is headed. For example, if you're meeting with a school official, are you asking for a switch to all-organic food, the addition of one vegetable dish and one piece of fresh fruit for every meal, or just the option of dried fruit in the vending machine? Or perhaps what you want is for the official to form a committee to look into the food issue, or to apply for a grant to improve school food, or to empower you and your committee to do more research with support from the school. Whatever you're looking for, get clear about it before you go in.

STAND IN THEIR SHOES. I do wonder sometimes, *When did it get so hard to be a mom?* Don't you think our kids' teachers are feeling the same way? And what about the principals? Can you imagine managing all of the new demands that children with allergies, ADHD, autism, and asthma must place on a school? Empathize with the other attendees, who will certainly have their own stories to share. And then collaborate on ways to work together to make *everyone's* lives easier!

END THE MEETING WITH A CLEAR PLAN FOR FOLLOW-UP. No matter how the meeting goes, you want the person you're meeting with to know that you'll be following up. Figure out your follow-up ahead of time or discover it spontaneously in the meeting—but either way, don't let the meeting fizzle to a close. Instead, one of you should say something like "We'll be calling you in a week to see what kind of progress you're making" or "We'll get back to you as soon as we've got the answer to that question you had." Follow your instincts—just make sure you don't end this step without making plans for the next one.

DON'T GIVE UP! You may get a terrific response first time out of the box—but you easily might not. Don't be discouraged—change takes time. Remember why you're doing this—to make a better world for your kids and to keep them healthy down the road—and you'll find the patience that has sustained you through all your other Mama tasks. Talk with your group about what your next step might be: finding more facts, broadening your group, appealing to another school official, making the issue public, raising the issue at a schoolwide meeting. It may take awhile to find the option that works best, but one thing I've learned is that there always *is* another option. If you can't accomplish something one way, you often can get it done in another. Think like a toddler! Do they *ever* take "no" for an answer?

Make Some Changes in Your Local Grocery Store

Does your store offer the rBGH-free milk that you've decided to try? If so, thank them! If not, make a request. Are you longing for an organic section that they just don't have? Can you find bread, cereal, and muffins *without* high-fructose corn syrup? If your grocery knows there's a demand, it might well respond. You can use the previous set of suggestions—find allies, set up a meeting, plan a meeting, etc.—to work with the grocery store as well. Don't forget to add that you have highlighted their work to the press. A little added PR exposure does wonders for helping people do the right thing!

Write a Letter to the Editor

Do not be intimidated by this. Remember, journalists are people just like you and me. Some have young kids with autism, some have kids with allergies, some have a mom with Alzheimer's or a brother with testicular cancer. There is hardly a family in the country that isn't dealing with some health issue. So write to them as you would write to a friend or a colleague. Keep it short and sweet and to the point. Choose one of the issues that is most personal to you. Begin with an opening sentence that summarizes your concern, follow up with three to five key points, and conclude with a brief sentence that serves as a call to action.

I've only made a few suggestions here. Use them as a starting point and go beyond them if necessary. One thing I've found: the first step is usually the hardest. At least it was for me. But once you take even the tiniest baby step, whether it's cutting out the blue yogurt or calling a friend to tell her about the Southampton Shocker, the rest seems to follow naturally because you're figuring things out as you go. There is such inspiration that comes in doing something that feels *so good* that you will develop your own momentum.

So don't worry too much about doing things right or even doing them well. Just do *something* and allow the rest to follow. I can't tell you how many meetings I attended with a baby on my hip and a sippy cup in my bag.

Was it my first choice to do the meeting that way? Not at all. But usually, it was my only choice. I schlepped more bottles, crayons, and diaper bags into professional offices than you can imagine. And you know what? I honestly think that it helped my cause. I mean, what option did I have? Waiting until my kids were all in college? Or doing it in what I now fondly refer to as "Mama gear"?

Taking action wasn't always easy—but I was always glad I'd done it. I'm willing to bet that once you figure out the first step *you* want to take, you'll be glad, too.

Holding Fast

As I began to find my voice and speak up about these issues that seemed so important for me and my family, I was so touched and comforted by the responses of people like Nell Newman, Robert F. Kennedy, Jr., and Erin Brockovich. If people of that caliber could believe in me, I thought, then I must be doing *something* right.

I'll always be grateful to Erin and Nell for publicly going on record in my support, putting their names beside mine on a contentious issue. Nell's team continues to help me get the word out about the hidden ways that our food affects our children's health. Erin spoke on my behalf in the *New York Times* article about me and connected me with nonprofits working to understand the dangers of environmental toxins. Even more moving to me was the way she shared her personal stories about her own struggles with these issues. Robert F. Kennedy, Jr., gave me my first platform to link genetic engineering and the allergy epidemic, which won credibility and attention for this issue. Their support and encouragement is a constant reminder that if you reach out with passion and sincerity, you will find people to lend their strength to your cause.

In that spirit, I'd like to share with you something quite personal, as you may encounter a similar response to your own efforts to change the way you feed your children. After all, food is such an intimate way of caring for your family. It makes sense that changing our relationship to it often makes our loved ones uncomfortable or even angry.

As I began to choose a different path from the one that I had been raised on, my family of origin remained distant, which I found very hard. At times, I felt as if I had been abandoned at sea. Losing the closeness I'd felt with my siblings and mom was hard extremely hard, as was the break with my dad.

I had always had a tough-love relationship with my dad. After all, he was a military man who had attended boarding schools as a kid and belonged to the Reserve Officers Training Corps (ROTC) in college. He was definitely a man of discipline. And when I began to make choices that diverged from his belief system, he took it personally, as if I was somehow judging the way that he and my mom had chosen to feed us. No matter how I tried, I couldn't convey that my choice was not a statement about how I was raised, but simply an effort to do as much as I could to protect the health of my kids.

As my dad and I diverged, I drew on my own version of the discipline I'd learned from him, working as hard as I could to convince him that this wasn't some "eating disorder" that my family had suddenly developed, but a reasoned, intelligent commitment to a healthy choice for my kids. I didn't make much headway though. My father simply did not want to acknowledge the information that I was unearthing.

At first, I wondered if he just didn't understand that the box of mac 'n' cheese that my brother so loved as a kid wasn't the same as the one sold for *my* kids. The food had changed and new ingredients had been added that had never been tested for safety. I told him that our food should be clearly labeled so that we had a clear choice about what to feed our kids. But, ever respectful of authority, he said that if the FDA found food safe, then it was safe. Period.

As I learned more about organic foods, I tried to explain to my father that these products contained fewer chemicals, pesticides, antibiotics, and hormones. His response was that they were just another marketing scheme. I even had my kids try to explain it to him. He told them that he didn't want to hear about it.

I tried to talk money. Given his disciplined work ethic, he'd always understood that. I explained that organic food cost more because the government didn't subsidize organic crops the way that they subsidized the conventional, genetically modified ones. Not only were there very few handouts and taxpayer dollars going to the organic farmers, but these same farmers also had to pay extra fees to prove that their products did not contain the chemicals, hormones, and antibiotics contained in conventional foods. I shared how in Europe, organic food is simply called "food" and that it's genetically modified food that must be labeled. My father was unmoved.

His face changed, though, when I mentioned the likelihood that the milk, soy, and corn found in everything from the Kraft box to the cans of Dr. Pepper he'd always enjoyed had been genetically altered by Monsanto.

"You know," he said, "I am just not sure that I buy all of this. I'm a Monsanto shareholder and I just read their annual report cover to cover. They don't mention any of this."

Of all the responses I had expected, this one wasn't on the list, and it stopped me dead in my tracks. Somehow I managed to look my father straight in the eye and say, "And I'm sure that Philip Morris's annual report didn't disclose that cigarettes could cause lung cancer either, Dad."

As I sadly turned away, I realized that I would never be able to convince my dad of a truth that was too inconvenient for him to hear.

To this day, my father is still a Monsanto shareholder. But I can't stop speaking out about Monsanto, or that mac 'n' cheese, or any other issue that is important to me and to our children's health. Given how contentious the issue became, my dad and I had to agree to disagree.

You, too, may encounter seemingly insurmountable odds in your efforts to protect your children. No matter where that resistance comes from, it will hurt, but this is where you have to trust your Mama Instinct, listen to your heart, and hope that those who are resisting will one day understand. I pray that my dad will understand, too.

So don't stop moving forward. For a while, you may feel as though you're taking two steps forward, one step back. And there may be some personal heartache along the way. But when you look your little ones in the eye, you will find your voice and take a stand for them. We are their voices. And we must have the courage to stand up for them, whatever the odds or however powerful the opposition might be.

Our reward will come years down the road, when our children ask what we did to make it better for them, and we get to answer:

> I bought chemical-free milk; I cut the powdered orange packet in half; I learned how to steam a chicken breast or make cinnamon toast. I taught my friends about it, so their kids could be safe, too. I urged our leaders to place the same value on your life that has been placed on the lives of children around the world. And I did it all because I love you.

8

THIS IS A CARROT

I won't lie to you: When I first realized how much "junk" was in my family's diet, I felt completely overwhelmed. And the more I learned about the problems with genetic engineering, processed foods, potential allergens, artificial colors, and other possible dangers, the more overwhelmed I felt.

Now, however, two and a half years after Tory's initial diagnosis, I look back with relief. Although I often *felt* daunted by the changes I planned to make, my family and I actually came through the transition pretty well. I didn't need to imitate Martha Stewart or turn into someone who cultures her own yogurt out of fresh goat's milk. Nor did my kids need to turn into little angels clamoring for bean sprouts and organic celery sticks. Perhaps most important, our shift to a healthier diet didn't require taking out a second mortgage or even cutting back on our few luxuries, like a night out and movie rentals. Much to my relief, it turned out there were some relatively simple, easy, and low-cost ways to lose the junk.

As we gradually got rid of the blue yogurt and the bright-orange mac 'n' cheese, we made some important gains as well. I could see that my kids were going to bed faster, for one thing. Before we switched to a healthier diet, we were always in for a minimum of half an hour and often as much as an hour of nighttime struggles. After we cut out the additives and colors—some of which are actually called excitotoxins because they excite the brain—the kids were just a lot calmer.

Now, I'm not saying this is going to be true of every kid. Besides the environmental component of the chemicals and the diet, there's also the genetic piece. I'm sure there are some kids who can eat a tube of blue yogurt and go straight to bed afterward. But in our house, color theory made a difference.

It wasn't just the kids, either. Jeff and I would get used to eating our healthy home diet and then go out to dinner in a local restaurant—and then we'd both lie awake for an extra four hours! I'm not saying that a luxury meal isn't worth it, sometimes, but it's good to have that extra rest.

Not only at bedtime were my kids better behaved. I've seen that when they're eating a basically healthy diet—with time-outs for the friends' birthdays or the school pizza days or the other special occasions—my kids generally get along better, are more cheerful, more energetic, and better able to control their impulses. From my own personal observation, the Southampton experiment was absolutely correct: my kids seem more hyper when they've ingested that chemical cocktail and they all seem calmer when they haven't. Their teachers have noticed the difference, too, commenting that my kids are paying better attention in school and are better able to handle the ups and downs of a kid's stressful day.

Sure, there are plenty of doctors who will say this is anecdotal at best (make sure to do a quick Google search on their name along with the word "disclosure" to see who might be paying them to talk!). My suggestion? Let's have these doctors babysit our kids for an afternoon on a day that they've attended a birthday party and loaded up on the artificial colors and preservatives in every bite they took.

Again, I can see the difference in Jeff and myself as well as in the kids. We're both more even-tempered, less "hyper and crashy," more able to ride out the stresses and storms of a four-child family and two very busy parents. Of course, I'm still a coffee junkie—and to be honest, I don't ever intend to give up my caffeine. Jeff and I still enjoy our nachos and beer when we go out for our weekly date night. But most of the time, our healthy diet pays off in energy, calm, and emotional resources—all worth their weight in gold to any parent.

You've already heard about the wonderful changes in Colin's personality, how a whole bubbly, happy side of him began to appear once dairy products weren't making his tummy and his head hurt. My other kids have undergone similar Jekyll-and-Hyde-like changes, depending on what they're eating.

For example, Lexy, my oldest, used to get hot lunch at school once or twice a week. Before we switched our eating habits, I used to think of it as my own personal little crutch: for $2.50, I could get out of packing one more brown bag. And as any mom knows, it is the little things that matter and can take a load off.

As our healthy diet began to kick in, I realized that Lexy considered her hot lunch days to be a special treat and I didn't want to deprive her. We agreed that she could have one hot lunch a week, and we'd look at the menus together and pick one out. I tried to at least choose a day where she'd get a fruit cup or something that seemed halfway nutritious.

But still, on her hot lunch days, she'd be a real little monster by the time I picked her up. She'd pout, cry, yell, complain, and burst into tears—all over nothing. If you knew my sweet, sunny, helpful Lexy, you'd realize what a dramatic shift this was. Even she was aware of it, because when she *wasn't* in the throes of a terrible mood, she'd be horrified—and bewildered—by her own bad behavior. We likened her to a volcano eruption. She *couldn't* control herself; however much she wanted to, she just couldn't.

"Lexy," I asked her one day, "do you think you're acting this way because you had hot lunch today?"

Lexy glared at me as only a scornful six-year-old can. *"No,"* she said defiantly. "It's *not* because of that."

I couldn't really blame her. Hot lunch was her treat, and who wants to give up a special treat, especially when it's food? We all cling to our culinary comforts, and hot lunch was Lexy's.

But after three weeks of gently suggesting to her that hot lunch might be the culprit, I had had enough. "Lexy," I said finally, "I really notice that every week, the day you've gotten your hot lunch is the day you're in a really bad mood after school. I'm thinking that the chemicals in the food might be making your tummy or your head hurt, which tends to make you act angry and upset. So the next time you have hot lunch, let's do an experiment. If you can behave that afternoon when I pick you up, you can keep having hot lunch. But if you can't, then I think the hot lunches will have to go."

"Fine," Lexy said, glaring at me again. "I *will* behave. You'll see." But of course, she couldn't. How can anyone keep from pouting or lashing out when they're in pain?

Lexy is a smart girl, though, and she really didn't like acting out—no kid *likes* to act that way. And when Lexy realized herself how hot lunches were affecting her, she made her own decision to give them up. I was so proud of her that we hit the toy store to reward such a "smart choice"!

Working with my daughter, I learned so much about how our kids are often smarter than we give them credit for. If we teach them while we are teaching ourselves, they can surprise us by how willing they are to keep up with our changes. In fact, if I were going to leave you with only one lesson in this whole chapter, that would be it: *Respect the intellect of your children—teach them what you're doing and give them the respect of explaining what the problem is.* When you really teach your kids about food and diet—or anything else—they become empowered. Suddenly, they're making their own choices, and somehow, the battle goes away.

At least, that's in the long run. In the short run, you may be in for a tantrum or two! But I promise you, you'll see good results sooner than you think, and every good thing that happens will give you that much more energy to take the next step, and then the next one, and the one after that.

So let's get started! Here are my basic, simple, and easy-to-follow suggestions for helping your family switch to a healthier diet.

Getting Started

Because making the shift to a healthier kitchen was always such a daunting task to me, I'm going to help you make it as easy as possible to take those steps toward protecting the health and well-being of your children and your family. Think of me as your next-door neighbor, sharing secrets at the park. And remember—I'm no Queen of the Kitchen. I *have* been known to burn noodles!

The first step is realizing that each of us is going to make the journey in our own way. For some of you, the first step will be to turn a detective's eye on the labels at the grocery store and choose one type of additive to reject, such as aspartame or Yellow 5. In my case, I got rid of rBGH first, despite the FDA claims that it is safe.

You might prefer to begin by navigating your grocery store a bit differently. Once you learn that most of the processed foods are in the middle aisles, you may want to stick to the "fresh-food" perimeters of the store and shop along the edges.

Or maybe you'll choose to vote with your shopping cart, replacing Kraft mac 'n' cheese with an organic brand, or perhaps deciding to make your own dish by drizzling some olive oil over cooked macaroni (it actually takes *less* time than following the instructions on the package).

The important point is to remember that *you get to do this your own way.* I'm here to offer some concrete suggestions—you'll read plenty in a minute—but as you know the choice is yours. Do what seems as though it's going to work for you, avoid what seems like too much trouble, and trust in yourself and in the process. If there's one thing I've learned in the past two years, it's that change often happens slowly, and sometimes without our even realizing that it's happened. So let your shift from "junk" to "healthy" go at your own pace, along your own route, in your own style. That's the only way it's going to work for you anyway, so why not start out by feeling calm and in control?

Likewise, some of you will be able to navigate these changes on your own, while others will want the support of friends and family. Pick a girl-friend who also has a kid addicted to blue yogurt so that you can go through it together. When you have someone to share the stories with, you will find that they can be pretty hilarious! Or if you have a sister across the country who wants help breaking her kids' addiction to cans of ravioli, share some of the tips found in this section. It will feel so good to be helping the people you love. And if you need additional suggestions (say, for example, that your dad is having a hard time getting his head around some of this), then study up using the Resources section at the back of the book (and enlist the help of your mom!).

Sometimes change happens quickly, sometimes at a snail's pace—but stick with it, just as you had to do when you were teaching your baby how to eat solid foods. Remember how messy that was? So give yourself some slack and realize that this change will probably be equally messy.

I feel honor-bound to warn you that these changes don't always come easy. Your immediate family may jump onboard right away, but some people in your life—friends or relatives—may roll their eyes at you or challenge your logic or even dismiss your efforts as "too fussy" or "out in left field." Sometimes, a cheese-and-cracker-eating grandfather or a Diet Coke–drinking grandmother is going to find these truths too inconvenient and will give you grief every step of the way, especially if they choose to see your new commitment to health as a veiled comment on the food that *they* served *you* growing up. Or you may have a sister-in-law who tells you that your children will be social outcasts, because their lunch-boxes don't contain the same levels of chemicals, additives, and preservatives as some of their classmates.

Take a deep breath and remember that food is an intimate thing. *You* know you're not doing this to make a point, or to put anyone down, or even to convince anyone else of the rightness of your actions. You're only trying to protect your health and the health of your loved ones. Keep reminding yourself of that central fact, and that will help make all the changes seem worthwhile. You just want chemical-free kids, like the moms in Europe have. So just like a toddler, don't take "no" for an answer!

So here we go! My first suggestion is a little lifesaver I discovered known as the *80–20 rule.*

The 80–20 Rule, *or* Moderation in All Things!

Hey, we're living in the real world, here, not in a cave. We don't have the time, energy, or resources to grow our own organic vegetable garden or tend to the flocks. Our kids go to birthday parties where cupcakes are served—they aren't any less interested in scarfing them down just because *you* now know that they're really high-fructose-corn-syrup bombs loaded with blue icing.

"Well," you think, "at least there'll be a healthy lunch first"—and then you learn that the party's being held at a pizza palace, which serves up affordable pizza, but at what cost?

I know we live in a crazy-busy world, where you need to grab and go, but those so-called convenience foods can make your life less convenient in the long run, if the price for all those chemicals is temper tantrums, endless bedtime battles, and pediatric bills.

Now, as you've heard, my own family was 100 percent dependent on these conveniently inconvenient foods, so how in the world was I going to wean them off? I mean, Colin's addiction to blue yogurt made him seem like my own little junkie, not to mention John's love of pizza, and Lexy's attachment to her once-a-week hot lunch. Thank goodness Tory was so little that she'd never been aware of anything other than the clean food I started her on as a one-year-old.

But I didn't want my other kids to have to go cold turkey. First, I wanted to spare them the withdrawal pangs. Second, and more selfishly, I wanted to spare *myself* the difficulties! I had come to depend on convenience foods to make my life easier—and as I keep saying, I couldn't cook.

In a perfect world, maybe we could all take the time to make everything from scratch with the most wholesome ingredients. In a perfect world, I could rest easy in the knowledge that every bite I put into my kids' mouths was made from ingredients produced by a local farmer who cared about my kids as much as I do. But I don't live in that world, and I'm willing to bet that you don't, either.

So what's a busy mom to do?

We follow the 80–20 rule (or at least this is our *ultimate* goal):

> If 80 percent of what we give our kids is healthy—free of additives, preservatives, artificial color, aspartame, MSG—then for the other 20 percent we, and they, get a free pass.

How does this work in practice?

Let's start with school. Your kids have five days of school each week, right? So try to reduce their exposure to the chemical cocktail on four out of every five school days. On the fifth day, let them have hot lunch if they want it. Or a cupcake. Or some other kid-friendly treat. In other words, don't make the *perfect* the enemy of the *good*. Don't you *need* a break from managing your kitchen, making school lunches, and trying to monitor this whole mess? I know I do! So give yourself a huge pat on the back for cranking out those four healthy lunches—80 percent of the lunches your kid ate that week—and take a break for the fifth lunch (there's the 20 percent).

Now, if you're like I was in 2006 and you've just read that last couple of pages, I can guess what you might be thinking: *80–20! I can't imagine even getting as far as 10 percent of their diet cleaned out and healthy! Have you seen my fridge, my life, my chaos? Our diets right now are 100 percent junk.* Right about now, the thought of trying to change your kids' diet may seem so overwhelming that you may just want to throw in the towel.

But if you've realized your kids have allergies, or discovered that artificial colors are making them hyper, or just plain gotten upset at the thought that there's so much *junk* out there (especially in what's supposed to be our "healthy" food!), then giving up isn't really an option, is it? So let's turn that 80–20 rule around. Let's call it the 20–80 rule, 20 percent healthy and 80 percent junk, or even the 10–90 rule, or even, if you're completely freaked out, the 1–99 rule. Let's start by changing *one* thing, just *one single thing* in your cupboards, fridge, or kid's lunch.

You can do that, right? You can always change just *one* thing. Right now, decide that that's *all* you have to change, just one thing, even if you've got 100 percent of the junk in your fridge and cupboards like I did. So what change would you like to make? A switch from conventional milk to organic or at least rBGH-free milk? *One* different snack a week for your five-year-old? (See the suggestions starting below.) *One* colored item replaced with a natural one, say, blue yogurt switched into plain white yogurt with your kid's choice of honey, raisins, apples, or bananas for sweetness? Or what about simply trading the multicolored Goldfish crackers for the orange ones?

You might also ask, "What *one thing* does our family consume the most of in any given week, like milk, that I'd like to focus on?" and then change *that*. One change, but far-reaching consequences. Or, if that sounds too much like a battle, pick something trivial that no one will notice and change *that*. Just get started—the rest will come in time.

Make that change. Take a deep breath. Commit perhaps to making only one change each week. Or one change each month. Pick something that seems small enough, and easy enough, that you can actually picture yourself doing it. And that won't break the bank.

Liking the idea but having a hard time imagining how to implement it? Here are some suggestions to get you started:

INSTEAD OF:	CHOOSE THIS!
Kool-Aid	Pure juice with water and sugar to taste
Jell-O	Knox unflavored gelatin mixed with pure fruit juice
Cheetos	Fritos or Natural Cheetos
Flavored oatmeal packets	Plain oatmeal with a spoonful of sugar, jam, or jelly
Tang	Orange juice

INSTEAD OF:	CHOOSE THIS!
Fat-Free Miracle Whip	Original Miracle Whip
M&M's	Chocolate chips
Lender's Blueberry Bagels	Lender's Cinnamon Raisin Bagels
Swiss Miss Milk Chocolate Cocoa Mix	Swiss Miss Chocolate Sensations Cocoa Mix
Froot Loops and Lucky Charms	Crispix and Cracklin' Oat Bran
Hawaiian Punch	Minute Maid Fruit Punch
NutraSweet/Equal	Sugar or stevia (natural no-calorie sweetener)
Diet Coca-Cola/sodas	Original Coca-Cola/sodas
Hershey chocolate candy bar	Ghirardelli chocolate candy bar
Imitation vanilla (vanillin)	Pure vanilla extract
Mello Yello	7Up (not diet)
Kraft Macaroni & Cheese mix—orange	Kraft Macaroni & Cheese mix—White Cheddar
Duncan Hines Devil's Food Cake mix	Duncan Hines Dark Chocolate Fudge Cake mix
Chocolate chip cookies	Sugar cookies
Prepackaged noodles with powder mix	Noodles with butter/olive oil
Prepackaged mix of rice	Plain rice with salt/spices added
Lowfat ice cream	Original ice cream
Strawberry ice cream	Vanilla ice cream with your own toppings!
Blue yogurt	Plain yogurt—add your own toppings

Then start to think about the 80–20 rule at mealtimes. We are not purists, we don't grow our own veggies (though given the recent sky-rocketing food prices, maybe we should). We are busy moms with picky kids! So start to think in terms of four out of five on their plates. Initially, if your house is at all like mine, you're going to look at your kids' plates and see Dinosaur Chicken Nuggets, glowing orange mac 'n' cheese, and bright-blue yogurt. "Wow," you think to yourself, "where do I start?"

Start with the 80–20 rule, or turn it around and make it 20–80. And pick *one thing*. If you serve five things for dinner, divide them into four plus one. For you and your kids, it may seem too much to change every-thing all at once, so cut yourself a break on four items (the 80 percent), and replace that fifth one (the 20 percent) with a chemical-free option. For example, replace that pot of blue yogurt with a piece of string cheese. Even if you can't initially afford the rBGH-free kind, you are taking all the important starter steps toward reducing your kids' exposure to all of those chemicals.

Once you're comfortable with 20–80, step it up to 40–60: *two* chem-free choices, and three items from your former diet. When the time is right, you can flip those stats to 60–40, and before you know it, you'll be up to 80–20: four healthy choices, and one free pass. Congratu-lations!

Anyone who's read the rest of this book knows that I completed this process at a snail's pace myself. My first step, back in January 2006, was giving Tory Safeway's organic baby food. The other kids didn't get so much as an extra carrot. In the spring of 2006, I started buying rBGH-free milk and more veggies for my other kids. Finally, that fall, I figured out how to dump most of the processed foods in favor of chem-free choices. But we have never stopped following the 80–20 rule, unless a kid's allergies were so severe that eating a forbidden food made him or her sick. Otherwise, my kids got their pizza slices, ice-cream cones, fast-food treats, and hot lunches. They just didn't get them every day.

Here is one final bonus. Once you get to that happy 80–20 place, where four out of five things your kid eats every day are healthy, your kids themselves will begin to taste the difference between the real food and the chemical-laced ones. Eventually, even to your kids, the real food is going to taste better—and your battle will be won. So keep your eyes on the prize!

Okay, now that you've got the 80–20 principle in your head, here are some other specific ways that you can start to implement it.

Reject rBGH

This one might initially appear to be a bit more expensive, but it's got the advantage of being subtle: it's unlikely that your kids will notice the switch from regular milk to rBGH-free milk. Happily, such major chains as Safeway, Publix, and Kroger are now routinely providing rBGH-free milk, as is Starbucks. You can usually also find rBGH-free cheese, yogurt, and ice cream if you look. Kraft has an rBGH-free product line.

If your kids are like mine, a huge percentage of their diet comes from milk and cheese. So if you do switch to healthier milk, you'll knock your 80–20 ball out of the park. You'd probably be well on your way to earning Mother of the Year.

And if you need some extra motivation on this one? Just think of the cancer and udder pus! (For more on the dangers of rBGH-laden milk, see chapter 4.) To strengthen your argument to any naysayers out there, keep an eye on your pediatrician bills and all of the costs associated with ear infections, eczema creams, and antibiotics, as you may find yourself saving some money there, too.

Cut the Colors

After we cut out the rBGH in our house, we went on to lose the fluorescent rainbow of colors. Of course, we had to do this slowly, since they seemed to be *everywhere:* in the neon orange mac 'n' cheese that I served up for dinner, in the bright-blue yogurt that the kids had for breakfast, and in the glowing yellow Goldfish crackers that were in their lunch boxes. Maybe those "charms" in their cereal weren't so lucky after all!

We took it step by step. Here is exactly how I weaned my kids—and myself—from that processed mac 'n' cheese that reminded me so fondly of my brother, who had devoured it during our childhood:

1. *Switch from "orange" to the packaged "white cheddar" variety.* Since initially I was still hooked on the convenience mentality and having everything come in one box, I made the initial switch from the bright orange to the white version. Still lots of preservatives in the powder, no doubt, but at least we'd lost the fluorescence.

2. *Only use part of the powder in the package.* Following my 80–20, or rather my 20–80, rule, I literally took a scissor and snipped off one-fifth of the package. I figured at least they were getting a *few* less chemicals. Then I started tossing out half of the powdered package. Then, eventually, I used none of it.

I have to be honest: the whole process took a while. First I had to get the kids used to the idea that their noodles didn't have to be bright orange, then the idea that they could be *just orange,* then to the idea that they could be a *faint* orange . . . then, finally, they agreed that noodles were supposed to be just white.

3. *Cook up some noodles and then drizzle them with olive oil. Grate some rBGH-free cheddar or Parmesan onto the top.* For extra time-saving, get one of your kids to help you grate the cheese—it's a remarkably kid-friendly chore if your grater isn't too sharp. Or buy a few of those little graters where you insert the cheese and turn the plastic handle and let each kid add his or her own cheese, which adds a colorful flair to the colorless meal. And make sure to teach them *why* and *how* they are doing remarkable things to protect themselves from chemicals—just like the kids in Europe!

For yogurt, we also took it step by step. As we weaned ourselves from blue yogurt, I returned to buying the plain white kind. To keep my kids from having a complete conniption, here's what we did:

1. *Give them colored sprinkles to add.* Yes, those rainbow-colored sprinkles that are *also* loaded with red, yellow, and blue dye. I let them add as many as they wanted to until they got used to the fact that their yogurt was white. (*"Mom!* It's *white!"*) This step took a few weeks, but when the kids finally stopped commenting on their yogurt's surprising whiteness, we moved on to step 2.

2. *We ran out of sprinkles.* Oops! All gone! How did that happen? Hey, kids, I know, let's find another way to keep our yogurt from being boring. Now the kids had the options of raisins, blueberries, nuts (for those who could do nuts), brown sugar, syrup, honey, jelly . . . you get the idea. And kids love the idea of concocting things themselves.

Initially, I didn't police the amount of jelly scooped into the yogurt too closely. If you want to win at the healthy eating game, you pick your battles wisely, and my first concern was to break their addiction to the chemicals in the blue stuff. Eventually, I began to regulate, but not until white yogurt with natural toppings was the normal order of the day.

We didn't go cold turkey with our Goldfish crackers either. First the multicolored kind, then the orange kind, then the uncolored kind (you can find them, and they're still goldfish shaped), and finally, the ones made out of pretzels. Call it the coward's way out or consider it the realpolitik of the kitchen—but my motto is, avoid as many battles as you can! And you *know* how to wean a kid—you did it when you were nursing, you did it with the bottle, you did it with the sippy cup. You're a parent. You can do this!

If you're trying to go color free, look for alternatives that don't use numeric codes to define colors. If you're taking it slow, start by opting out of Yellow 5, a.k.a. tartrazine (since Kraft doesn't use it in England, why should we?).

And for extra added fun with your older kids, help them identify that little pound sign and then enlist their help in perusing every single item in your grocery cart or on your kitchen shelves to find it. Your kids may find that they have just as much fun helping you throw out or avoid buying those colored foods as they used to have in eating them.

Avoid the Artificial

If a label includes "artificial ingredients" or "imitation" in the description, put it back on the shelf. And here's another good rule of thumb: when reading ingredients and labels, less is usually more. The shorter the ingredient list on the side of the box, the better. You're also looking for shorter words *in* the ingredient list.

A third rule is the "Grandmother Guideline": if your grandmother didn't have it in her kitchen, you probably don't want it in yours. So if you come across an ingredient that you can't even pronounce, chances are that Grammy would not have had it sitting in her cupboard or on her counter. Probably it was made in a lab either to preserve it on the shelf (got to wonder what *that* does inside of you) or to make it more appealing to your kid.

So not only do you want a shorter ingredient list, you also want shorter words. Words you can actually pronounce. A great test of this is to make sure that your kids can pronounce the words, too. In fact, one of the most fun ways you can help make this transition with your kids is to turn them into mini-detectives. Make it as big a deal as you like—and then ask them to help you track down any words that are too long, too weird, or too full of numbers. They will *love* learning about all of this, and you can all have fun making up ways to pronounce those multisyllabic words that even *you* can't read.

Cereal Killers

It's a good bet that the cereals that contain name-brand cookies and similar treats have dialed up the amount of artificial ingredients as well. So start by nixing the name brands—but tell your kids why! Say something like, "Honey, there are too many chemicals in that cereal that are dangerous for you. Mommy loves you *too* much to feed you chemicals, which is why we have to choose a new cereal."

Kids will get that. They don't want to get sick.

An extra added bonus is that here is one place where going healthier is actually cheaper. You'll save more than a few pennies if you stop purchasing those chemically loaded name brands. According to Marion Nestle at the Department of Nutrition and Food Studies at New York University and author of *Food Politics,* only twenty cents of every dollar spent on food actually goes to the food producer. Which means that the remaining eighty cents goes toward the packaging, labeling, and marketing of that particular item. Why should you subsidize those big companies' marketing, when all you want is the food? (The *twenty cents'* worth of food!)

So ditch the box and grab the bag—you know, the ones on the bottom shelf at the grocery store that they really don't want you to focus on? Did you know that leading brands pay top dollar to get their products in the best position on grocery store shelves? Since the bag guys don't have the economic muscle of the box boys, the cheaper choices can usually be found below.

If you really want to pay for *just* the food, then hit the bulk aisles that are starting to pop up in Safeway and Kroger as well as in the organic grocery stores, and have your kids help you scoop the cereal, raisins, or sugar out of the bins themselves. Your grandmother would be proud!

By the way: If supermarkets and grocery stores only have an aisle or two set aside for "Healthy Foods," then what do you call the rest of the food in the store? Just asking.

Chemicals in a Can

If you haven't given your kids soda yet, my advice is, don't start. Think of this drink as "chemicals in a can," and you'll be hard-pressed to hand it over to your kids. Tell *them* that it is chemicals in a can, and, as with the cereal, explain that you love them too much to feed it to them. You might try explaining to your kids how bad the chemicals are for them and then asking them what advice they would give to you—or to a hypothetical mommy who loves her children. Sometimes when kids solve a problem on their own, they're quicker to invest in the right answer than when we just hand it to them.

If you've read chapter 6, you already know that Coca-Cola makes U.K. versions of Coke and Diet Coke that *don't* contain some of the worst of the cancer-causing chemicals. It still makes me crazy that we don't have that option here, especially because, as a sleep-deprived mother of four, I would have to say that I had an addiction to my Diet Coke that I now have to satisfy entirely with coffee. Not to mention that I was starting to see Rumsfeld's face on every can of aspartame-laden diet soda that I picked up!

So while we break our own dependencies, let's not get our kids hooked, either. You wouldn't want your kids to pick up a cigarette, so don't let them pick up a soda can, either. Try some smoothies instead:

1. Find juice that does not contain high-fructose corn syrup or artificial colors. If conventional juice is all you can find or afford, at least go color-free—ban the blue and red. Pour in a half cup for each kid, right into the blender.
2. Toss in some frozen fruit. Good choices include pineapples, peaches, strawberries, blueberries, and mangos, but experiment with your kids to see what they like best.
3. Add a half cup of milk for each kid, as well. You can use rBGH-free cow's milk, or for the milk allergic, try rice milk,

almond milk, or even coconut milk. (After you read chapter 3, you may want to avoid soy milk, which can raise your kids' estrogen levels and which may be allergenic.)

4. Add a few ice cubes and a banana, and buzz for 2 or 3 minutes.

If you're chronically pressed for time—and who among us is not?—you can mix up a big batch of smoothies and stick them in the door of the fridge to finish drinking tomorrow. If you throw in a few ice cubes when you reblend it, the kids won't know the difference. Or store them in the freezer. Your kids can eat them with a spoon or wait for them to melt. As you'll see below, I'm all about cooking it once, and then eating it twice!

Liquid Lunch

"Chocolate milk is soda pop in drag."

Those are the unforgettable words of the Renegade Lunch Lady, Chef Ann Cooper, who has been working to bring healthy school lunches to the lucky kids in California.

Bearing those artificial growth hormones in mind, I wasn't sure I wanted to add an extra dose of chemicals by "chocolate-ing" up the stuff. Sure, I could buy my kids organic chocolate milk, if I felt generous that day, but sometimes the budget just said no. Even when we had a few extra bucks in the bank, I found myself beginning to get annoyed at the price I had to pay for the organic version, which eventually led me to the point where I just stopped buying the stuff.

The result? Complete throw-down temper tantrums by my toddlers in the middle of the bagel store. Time for a new treat! That's how the smoothies came into our house (and the $1 toy bins at Target were also a lifesaver as a substitute for "treats.").

So if you're looking to make your 80–20 quota, consider switching from chocolate milk to fruit-and-ice smoothies. Your kids will still be tasting sweet, cool goodness—but you won't be giving them hormones and additives.

Next time you hesitate, just read the side of a container of chocolate milk mix and think of your grandmother. Words like those were probably only used by biochemists back in her day.

Juice Junkies

Now the juice industry (along with the cereal guys and the soda pop gang) are going to tell you that sugar and additives don't make your kids hyper. I'd love to test that theory out on these industry-funded experts: maybe we could lock *them* in a room with a bunch of kids who've just been given a red juice box and a bowl of sweet stuff and see, after an hour or two of this isolation, if they still reach that same conclusion.

Meanwhile, *you* can wean your kids off their sugar highs by applying the 80–20 rule: mix their juice with 20 percent water in order to cut the sugar. In all likelihood, your child won't even notice, but if your kid freaks, then take it slower: 90–10 or even 99–1. The important thing is to start the transition and then keep on making it, however long it takes.

Please remember, too, that this is one other crucial place where going healthier—say, with fresh fruit instead of the juice, and with water instead of the sweeter liquid—may actually be cheaper, because when you think about your yearly grocery budget, you are paying a king's ransom to have the juice put in those little boxes. Sure, they are convenient, but once again: eighty cents of every dollar you spend is going for the box, the straw, and the price of being placed on a toddler-high shelf! Those are marketing dollars aimed straight at your kids. You don't have to subsidize that!

If your kids absolutely prefer juice above all drinks, maybe load up on some big jugs of some all-fruit version—no additives, color, or high-fructose corn syrup—and pick up a few cool sippy cups, too. Then blend 80 percent of the juice with 20 percent water. Not only will you save money, you will head off the roller-coaster mood swings and late-afternoon temper tantrums as your kids consume less sugar and more nutrients.

Switching Snacks

I found that one of the hardest parts of my transition from "junked" to healthy was snacktime. As a mother of four, I was always on the fly. It was one thing to put healthy food on my kids' plates at mealtimes or even to pack them healthy lunches. But snacks were supposed to be easy! And we relied on the chemical cocktail more during snacktime than at any other.

As with everything else, I made the transition in a series of baby steps. Here are some of the little changes we made in our house.

Swimming in a Sea of Goldfish

Step 1: Replace the multicolored Goldfish crackers (you know, the green, red, and orange ones!) with the bright-orange Goldfish.

Step 2: Replace the orange Goldfish with the uncolored or pretzel versions.

From Chips to Dips

Our kids loved chips and I hated to deprive them. But I just couldn't stand to see them crunching those fluorescent orange deep-fried chemical compounds every day after school.

Now we occasionally have a bag of chips as a special treat, but mostly my kids dip crackers, rice crackers, or pretzels into ketchup, mustard, yogurt, or honey. Sure, there are chemicals in their dips, too, but far fewer than if they scarfed down a bag of chips. Remember, it's not a perfect world—but it can be a better one! I can also dream of the day that they ask for carrots and celery sticks to crunch on instead of chips, can't I?

Make Your Own Snackpacks (And Get Your Kids to Help!)

Step 1: Tell your kids why you're not buying the prepackaged versions anymore: too many chemicals and you love them too much to give them food that's bad for them.

Step 2: Get creative and make your own snackpacks following the 80–20 rule. Enlist the help of your kids. I mix four healthy choices into the bag, and make the fifth one the bonus feature! For example: raisins, nuts (if you can swing it in an allergy-free house), some pretzels, some little crackers (from a box with a short list of ingredients that you can pronounce), and—as the bonus—maybe a chocolate chip or two (or if you're like me and hate throwing out food, you may want to use up the candy-coated cereal here or the M&M's you still have or the yogurt raisins that you didn't realize were coated in rBGH-laden dairy).

Step 3: Make a dozen or so little bags—with your little ones helping—and stash them for the week. Done! Give yourself a hug!

Minutes Matter

At mealtimes, I don't need to tell you: minutes matter. Every mom knows how valuable those minutes, even seconds, are, when it comes to the witching hour at five o'clock. All hell can break loose at any moment!

So one of the best investments you can make in your new healthy-snack life is to spend $3.99 for an apple slicer. In fact, if you've got more than one kid, buy them each their own—you can find one in almost any grocery store with the cooking utensils. Your kids will love pressing it into a fresh apple and creating eight perfect slices, and you will be more inclined to serve up an apple because this gets rid of the time-consuming annoyance of having to slice it up yourself. (As I keep saying, we're all busy!)

By the way, it works on pears, too. And don't you love the idea that your kids are helping to make their own snacks?

For extra snacktime fun, you can use those eight apple pieces to play a math game with your kids. They're great for reviewing fractions!

Frozen Fruit

Speaking as a woman on a budget, I know how much more fruit seems to cost than all those packaged foods. Even given that 80 percent of the price of those snack foods goes to pay for packaging, it still seems cheaper to buy juice boxes and fruit rollups than to shell out for fresh apples, pears, and bananas, let alone strawberries, blueberries, and mangos.

But if you think about what your doctors' bills and meds are running you, fruit might just come to seem more economical in the long run. When your kids eat fresh fruit, they're avoiding those artificial colors and chemicals, and they're consuming those crucial nutritional building blocks that the fake foods don't contain. And since fruit is prepackaged in its own skin, you avoid paying the 80 percent of every dollar that goes toward the marketing of those chemical packages.

So how could I find an affordable way to get more fruit into my kids' diets? I hit the frozen foods aisle. What a wonderful discovery: frozen fruit is much cheaper than the fresh stuff. And little hands love grabbing those frozen blueberries, strawberries, or pineapple chunks straight from the bag. Frozen fruit is also a great substitute for ice cream that contains growth hormones. (Yes, you can buy rBGH-free ice cream, but it tends to be more expensive, alas.)

If you want to feel like a chef—and who doesn't—you might help your kids mix up a little bit of that white yogurt and some brown sugar, syrup, jelly, or honey. Then drizzle the mixture across the top of the frozen fruit and you've got something that's *almost* as much fun as an ice-cream sundae, but without the sugar rush, the chemicals, or the crash that inevitably comes two hours later. Nothing fancy, everything is totally homemade, and what an incredible job you have just done in cutting the chemical exposure in your kids' diet! Did you just earn Mother of the Year?

Baked to Order

Here is where we have to think like the French moms do. They don't buy prepackaged bread, loaded with preservatives, that has been shipped in from who knows where on a truck. They buy bread from the bakery.

Sure, a trip to the bakery aisle at your local grocery store isn't as romantic as say, strolling through some artsy district in Paris and picking up a baguette. But chances are that the fresh loaf of bread that you buy in the bakery section of Safeway has fewer preservatives in it than the prepackaged stuff. And, as Marion Nestle taught us, you'll be paying for the bread, not the packaging. In other words, you'll be saving money, avoiding chemicals, and doing so much for your kids with just this simple switch.

Of course, you have to pay attention, because bakery bread doesn't have a long shelf life. How could it, since it doesn't contain the chemical additives and preservatives that would otherwise keep it from going bad? Just like the bread our grandmothers knew, it can actually get stale or moldy. We've so loaded our foods with chemical additives and preservatives that many of us are no longer used to the simple fact that *real* food spoils.

Sure, the concept of preserving food on a shelf sounds good. But what are those preservatives doing to us once they get inside of our bodies? Or inside the bodies of our kids?

Mealtime Marvels

Okay, so now that we've got some snacks and treats lined up, what about the three squares? If you're like most moms I know—myself included—you rely on a few basic staples to get you through the week. In our house, that was dinosaur-shaped chicken nuggets, bright-orange mac 'n' cheese, blue yogurt, and packaged cereal. Heaven help me, I thought those choices *were* healthier than Happy Meals.

In a moment, I'm going to lay out some suggestions for seven days' worth of meals and snacks. But first, let me talk you through some of the new staples I worked out for me and my family—things I could whip together ahead of time on weekends or quickly during the week while still tending to four kids and a home-based business. I'll also share some of the principles that guide me through my kitchen—and keep me sane.

Cook It Once, Eat It Twice

There is hardly a mother on the planet who doesn't struggle with the task of getting her kids to eat in the manic and busy world in which we now find ourselves. There never seems to be enough time to shop, much less cook, much less insist on all of the healthy options that you know are important.

So what's a mom to do? Simplify.

For example, if you decide on Monday that you are going to cook up chicken breasts (see Grammy Nuggets, on page 249), then make sure that you've got enough chicken in there for two meals. Feed your kids some of it tonight and then use the rest in their sandwich for school tomorrow, or wrap it up in a tortilla for dinner the following night. Sanity saver!

Same goes for dishes like the beans and rice on page 249. Make enough for two meals, then ladle those beans and rice straight into a tortilla for a Mexican combo for lunch tomorrow. I don't have time to cook. Do you? So when I do, I do it with efficiency. After all, I've got four kids and a full-time job and the last place I want to be is slaving away over a hot stove at the end of a long day.

Grammy Nuggets

I had to find something creative to replace those chicken nuggets (hey, at least they were made with white meat!) but this was a challenge. Finally, I decided on Grammy Nuggets. In no way do these things resemble Grammy, a dinosaur, or a nugget, but calling them by this name helped ease the transition.

Grab two or three chicken breasts (frozen is fine, and make sure you've got enough for two meals). Then put a few tablespoons of olive oil in a frying pan along with a shot of water; add the chicken. Let your five-year-old sprinkle some salt and pepper on while the eight-year-old sprinkles the garlic, put a lid over the top, and steam away. If you used frozen or thawed breasts, you may want to slice them up before putting them in the pan so that they will cook faster. Otherwise, use some kitchen scissors to cut through the partially steamed breasts as soon as you are able to—again, they'll cook faster. Then tell the kids that this is the way that Grammy made nuggets when she was a kid.

Texas-Style Rice and Beans

I love this staple, which is super-easy to make and can also involve the kids. Add rice and water to a pot—three times as much water as rice, and ideally, brown rice. Two of my four kids still won't touch brown rice, so I usually make white rice one night and brown another, and then do the 80–20 blend: 80 percent white rice for Colin and John; 80 percent brown rice for Lexy and Tory. It's as "perfect" as I get!

Bring your rice of choice to a boil, then reduce the heat and simmer for 20 minutes (or use the quick-cook rice, which is even faster). Get a can of whatever kind of beans you like—black, red, kidney, garbanzo—

rinse the beans, and toss them through the rice when it still has a few minutes to cook, so the beans have a chance to heat up.

Then let the kids spice it up. Grinding pepper is a hit in our house. You can also give them salt, garlic, or whatever they want to add.

You can brown up some ground turkey or beef to supplement this veggie staple, or add guacamole or salsa on top. For those of you without dairy allergies, try some grated cheese on top—and let the kids add that, too.

Sanity-Saving Staples

As I mentioned earlier, noodles are great. As you wean your kids and family off of the orange stuff, they will have a blast playing chef in the kitchen when you let them either drizzle some olive oil and sprinkle salt and pepper over the top or add some grated Parmesan (those little round graters are a big hit with eight-year-olds). You can kill off the boxes of noodles, tossing out the prepackaged powder and replacing it with this culinary excellence.

Tortillas are also a great staple that can be filled with anything. Sure, quesadillas are a fun choice, but who said that you can't spread PB&J into tortillas for those kids who can manage the peanut butter?

For another head fake, why not replace those frozen pizzas with English muffins topped with spaghetti sauce plus whatever other things little fingers might want to add? These are hits in our house because they actually take *less* time to prepare than a conventional frozen pizza since they are so small. Lose the chemicals, keep the kids!

Planning for Picky Eaters

Believe me when I say that I can so totally relate to the challenges of feeding little kids. Our house is chock-full of picky eaters. One only wants his bagels plain, the other only wants his crispy, almost burned and loaded with honey. A third goes into convulsions at the site of anything green, freaking out at the mere smell of broccoli (though, I have to admit, this is understandable). And while Tory, my fourth, *isn't* a picky eater, she *is* allergic to eggs.

So the task of suddenly taking away some of their most basic food items, the ones that had become my crutches for surviving motherhood, frankly terrified me. The last thing that I wanted was a temper tantrum at the dinner table. Hadn't my day been long enough?

But then again, I hated those ripping ear infections that had kept our house up for nights on end and the raw eczema that no prescription cream could seem to clear up and the sleepless nights that came with the worry of spreading the industrial-strength steroid ointment all over my boys.

I realized that I had to do *something*. So I threw open the kitchen cupboards and thought about my week. All seven days. Twenty-one meals and the snacks, at least a few a day . . .

And then I wrote down the following:

7 breakfasts
7 lunches
14 snacks
7 dinners

I went on to design the following meal plan for my kids, which I'm now going to share with you, the busy mom/dad/wife/jock/desk jockey who now knows that your bowl of cereal probably contains corn engineered at the cellular level to release insecticidal toxins as it grows, and that the milk poured onto that cereal has been produced with an artificial growth hormone that might cause breast and prostate cancer, not to mention what it does to the cows. This is for you, because, thank goodness, you are savvy!

But I know you're also busy. Don't worry. This won't be any harder than what you already do—and I promise it will be a whole lot healthier.

Your First Shopping Trip—Keep These on Hand as Staples, Too

  fresh fruit: bananas, apples, oranges

  frozen fruit

  unflavored applesauce

  bacon/sausage (opt for nitrate-free bacon if possible and
    unflavored sausages)

  bread/bagels/English muffins (look for high-fructose corn
    syrup [HFCS]–free)

  cereals (less is more . . . less box, less color, less corn! And
    grab the bags on the bottom shelf!)

  rBGH-free milk/yogurt

  jelly, honey, sugar, brown sugar, cinnamon

  olive oil (to replace cooking spray)

  fresh bread from your grocery's bakery (think like the French
    moms!)

  pretzels

  potato chips

  raisins, dried fruits

  rBGH-free cheese (or rice cheese/almond cheese to suit your
    allergy kid)

  bags of noodles

  carrots

  tomatoes

  tortillas

  deli meat (look for nitrate-free)

  chicken breast

  ground turkey/beef

  beans

  rice

Your gimme: always add half a piece of fruit to any meal. Wash it, and you're off to a great start. Sometimes a kid can eat the entire banana, but usually half an apple, a pear, or an orange works great. Better to stick with fruit that doesn't have a high water content, so don't overindulge in watermelon and cantaloupe, as they tend to absorb not only the water but the chemicals in the water, including the pesticides. And since fruit can get expensive (especially in the winter), I start with half of a piece so that I don't waste any. After all, no one, especially not a five-year-old, likes a leftover brown apple or soggy pear! Or I use frozen fruit, which is cheaper than fresh.

And ditch the cream cheese. Instead use a slice of real cheese. rBGH-free is best, but even cheese is a better choice than cream cheese, which is mixed with who knows what? Sure, there may be agonizing wails of betrayal and dismay, but they *will* get over it. (Mine did.)

Also Buy

> thermoses
>
> straws
>
> little Tupperware pots for yogurt and other snacks
>
> cool sippy cups with straws to replace the juice boxes (yeah, I know about the issue with plastics; we'll save that for another book!)
>
> a spiraling cheese grater that little hands can wind
>
> an apple corer—one per kid if you want help in the kitchen

Remember: Engage the kids. If they are part of the process, they will be much quicker at adapting!

Breakfast: Some General Principles

Opt Out

> conventional corn-flakey cereal, since it likely contains GM corn
>
> high-fructose corn syrup, since it is almost certainly derived from GM corn and might contain mercury

synthetic colors

conventional milk/yogurt

Pop-Tarts (sadly, they contain different ingredients than the
ones that we consumed as kids, and the new ones are
just loaded with chemicals and GM crops that it is best
to avoid)

Opt In

other unsweetened cereal that has *not* been genetically modified, including all other grains: wheat, bran, oats, rice,
etc.

bread that does not contain HFCS (put your little mini-
detectives to work in the bread aisle, as fortunately, bread
without HFCS is becoming increasingly more common,
or grab a fresh loaf from the in-store bakery)

cinnamon toast, sugar sprinkles

rBGH-free milk/yogurt/cheese

Seven Breakfasts

1. *Fruit, bacon, cinnamon toast using bread that is HFCS-free
(read the labels!).* Cinnamon toast became our leggo-my-Eggo
waffle substitute after I had to toss a few boxes of frozen waffles,
which I hadn't realized were chock-full of junk. So we mourned
that loss for a while until we came up with cinnamon toast to replace it. We sprinkled sugar and cinnamon onto the toast, cut it
into slices, and dipped it into syrup (initially, to get used to the
new idea; eventually we lost the syrup, too).

Now I know full well that the Sugar Police are going to come
screaming at me, but again, this is to ease that transition period.
So don't let the perfect be the enemy of the good. If this is what
you have to do to get your kid to eat a piece of toast instead of a
frozen waffle or Pop-Tart, then do what you need to.

2. *Half a banana, unsweetened oat cereal/rice cereal.* You can add sugar, honey, or brown sugar to make it interesting. You can even add sprinkles if necessary, and ignore those sirens from the Sugar Police. Remember to grab the bags off the bottom shelves in the grocery store or, to make your grandmother proud, shop out of the bulk bins in the health food aisles. Use rBGH-free milk, or rice milk, almond milk, or other milk substitute depending on allergies.

3. *Half a bagel (HFCS-free), smoothies made with the frozen fruit of your kids' choice.* To make smoothies, take a shot of pure fruit juice (remember, you don't want HFCS-sweetened), a banana, your choice of milk. If you can't find sweet juice that does not contain HFCS, buy unsweetened juice and add honey to sweeten it. I follow the lead of my mother-in-law on this one and add a shot of fish oil. That sounds so gross, but if your child does not have a fish allergy, it's a great source of Omegas and fat.

4. *Pancakes.*

5. *Dutch babies.* This is a puffy pancake, but with no ladling or flipping required. Now you *are* going to feel like a gourmet chef.

Obviously, this recipe is for those of you who don't have a kid with allergies. Preheat the oven to 450 degrees. In a bowl, mix together ¾ cup of milk (rBGH-free if you can swing it), ½ cup of all-purpose flour, ¼ teaspoon salt, 2 eggs. Grease either a pie dish or an 8-inch round or square baking pan. Pour the mixture into it, sprinkle some sugar on top (or chocolate chips) and then bake it for ten minutes. Pull out the puffy pancake when it is slightly brown on top and serve with fresh fruit.

6. *Fried eggs on a piece of toast with a piece of fruit.* A quick breakfast for those who are not allergic. My egg eaters often prefer hard-boiled eggs (which are great for the Cook It Once, Eat It Twice mentality as they can also serve as afternoon snacks).

7. *Scrambled eggs with bacon.* If you can swing mixing up a few eggs with rBGH-free milk (and maybe some cheese?) while

getting your kid to add a sprinkle of salt and pepper, you'll be in
great shape! Substitute plain oatmeal flavored with jelly, honey, or
sugar if one of your kids is allergic to eggs.

Now if your house is at all like mine, you may not get this much variation in a week. Two or three of these breakfasts may work just fine for
you and your kids, so stick with what works. Diversity is not a strength
in the diet of some of my gang, I must admit, but I do the best with what
I've got. If toast, a piece of fruit, and a slice of bacon work for your kids,
aim to use bread that doesn't contain high-fructose corn syrup (HFCS)
and you've taken a big step in reducing your kids' exposure to insecti-
dal toast!

Lunch: Some General Principles

In my house, the kids probably get more or less the same thing packed
for lunch most days. Sure, I wish I were more gourmet and creative, but
I have picky kids, a limited budget, and no time. What about you?

If you're like me, the variation in the lunchtime routine comes when
you alternate between yogurt pots or applesauce, and between deli meat
or a PB&J sandwich.

So how can we clean up those lunches?

When I first became concerned about corn and corn products, I
started reading ingredient labels to learn where that corn was lurking and
was astonished to find that even a lot of sliced breads contain high-
fructose corn syrup. As I learned more about HFCS, I realized that not
only was it a cheap alternative to sugar (you can learn more about the politics of this one from books listed in the Resources section), but it is also
a preservative, so it helps prevent bread from getting moldy on grocery
store shelves. Great for the profitability of the bread companies and the
stores, but how are our bodies supposed to process those chemicals?

As I continued to read labels, I learned that organic bread, by law, cannot contain HFCS, but I was loath to pay $4 for an organic loaf of bread given that my four kids can demolish an entire loaf in a single meal. So what's a mom to do?

Think like the French moms and hit the bakery section. That bread is fresh, and most likely made with ingredients that your grandmother had in her kitchen. Just be prepared to use it soon after you buy it, since the lack of chemicals means that yes, it can go bad—but that's a *good* thing! So, before you lament the fact that you can't afford organic, just take a few steps over to the bakery section and buy a nonorganic but bakery-made loaf there; you know, the bread that comes in the brown bag? And think of the Eiffel Tower!

Chances are that your kids will *love* the taste of this fresh bread. And if they don't, then just pack the deli meat without any bread—who says that the turkey has to be sandwiched between preserved slices? They can eat it plain. Your husband will probably have already polished off the bread anyway!

Another great substitute for HFCS bread is a package of tortillas. Why not whip up a PB&J (for you lucky non–allergy kid families) sandwiched between two circles? Look for local brands: they're less likely to be loaded with preservatives because they didn't have to travel as far to get to your kitchen.

Another easy first step, lose the colored yogurt pots and colored chips. That will go a long way to reducing the chemical cocktail.

To make this transition in our house, we found a few substitutions. Pretzels and some ketchup for dipping is one of the faves: it's interesting, it gives my kids something to do, and it piques the curiosity of fellow lunch mates. It's also chemical-free if you opt for organic ketchup, since the conventional stuff can contain corn in the form of high-fructose corn syrup. But honestly, even the regular ketchup is better than those artificially colored snacks, so compromise where you can and cut yourself a break.

Now, until we can get Kraft to remove the chemical additives from their Lunchable lines in the United States, the way that they have done for the kids in the United Kingdom, it's probably a good idea to monitor the Lunchables' intake. But the alternatives I suggest are just about as fast and probably less expensive!

Eight Lunches (I Went Overboard! Why Stick to Seven?)

1. *Deli meat on fresh bread, pretzels with ketchup/mustard, piece of fruit.* Do they really eat more than that anyway?

2. *Fresh bread with spaghetti sauce for dipping, rBGH-free cheese stick/string cheese, applesauce.*

3. *Salami, a piece of fresh bread, carrots, leftover noodles.* Leftover noodles with either olive oil or grated cheese—from dinner last night—are a great way to cook once and eat twice.

4. *PB&J on fresh bread, color-free potato chips, smoothie.* Put the other half of their breakfast smoothie in your kids' thermos (they can grab a straw from the lunch line).

5. *Piece of fruit and a pizza pie on an English muffin.* Top an English muffin with spaghetti sauce, rBGH-free cheese, and meat, veggies, or whatever you can get away with. Then sandwich the pizza pie with the other half of the English muffin on top. I love this one: it's the perfect chemical-free combo meal.

6. *Fresh bread deli sandwich, plain yogurt with toppings, pretzels.* Include a variety of toppings for the yogurt, like granola, raisins, or even chocolate chips.

7. *Tortilla pie.* Same as the English muffin pizza only you make it between two tortillas with spaghetti sauce and veggies and deli meat.

8. *Rice and beans.* A cook-once, eat-twice lunch. Add a side of salsa or guacamole for your little chef to stir in, and a piece of fruit.

As you will notice, each meal will go a long way toward reducing the amount of chemicals in your kids' lunch box. Sure, there are still going to be chemicals hidden in some of the items, but remember 80–20, and the fact that you have done a great job at reducing 80 percent of the chemicals usually found in kids' lunches.

Fourteen Snacks

This was one area where I really had to go cold turkey. No more snack-packs. At least not until the American corporations decide to remove some of these chemicals from our kids' foods the way that they already have overseas. So we had to set about making our own. And it really was pretty darned easy (just make sure that you load up on those Tupper-wares).

After all, if they're hungry, they'll eat it. And after school, what kid isn't hungry?

1. *Uncolored Goldfish crackers.* Let them swim in a Ziploc or throw them into a Tupperware tank. Either way. Done. Make seven snackpacks.

2. *Pretzels.* Same thing. Ziploc or Tupperware. Pack up seven little bags or bowls and you are done!

3. *Applesauce.* Sure, you can buy the individual pots (store a pack of spoons in your glove compartment), but it is much cheaper to buy the big jars and jar your own (like your grandmother would have done). Buy seven Tupperware pots and you're done.

4. *Cereal.* It's not just for breakfast anymore. I sometimes even include it in lunches, and definitely in snacks. A thermos is handy for storing rBGH-free milk, rice milk, almond milk—whatever suits your fancy and fits your AllergyKid. Remember to keep those spoons in the glove compartment.

5. *Fruit.* If they are hungry, they will eat it. Bananas, oranges, or apples actually travel best and survive the inevitable beating that fruit can take on the road. And if your kids are at all like mine, a bruised banana can send your five-year-old into conniptions!

(Don't tell the kids, but those bruised bananas are perfect for smoothies, so save them and freeze them for later.)

6. *Raisins and other dried fruit.* Great as an after-school savior for the kid who has low blood sugar levels as it provides an immediate boost in that department. I find the immediate fix of an afternoon snack pretty critical, especially for my boys, who rush through their lunches in order to toss a ball around with friends, leaving them unfinished at least half of the time!

7. *Potato chips.* Again, we are not here to make the perfect the enemy of the good. Potato chips have their own issues, we know, but if you are considering the whole chemical-cocktail effect, potato chips are at least the same color as the food that they are derived from.

8. *rBGH-free cheese sticks and crackers.* Again, the crackers may not be 100 percent clean, but we live in the 80–20 world, and this is a smart choice for a busy family, as it is much better than the multicolored, finger-staining (and digestive-staining?) corn chips.

9. *rBGH-free yogurt with your choice of toppings.* Top with honey, jelly, chocolate chips, cereal sprinkles, granola, brown sugar: endless possibilities! You are sure to find something to satisfy that toddler's taste. What about a scoop out of the frozen juice can in the freezer? Or a scoop out of the smoothie that you stocked in the fridge door?

10. *A slice of toast/English muffin/half a bagel.* Do what you can to avoid HFCS since chances are that it is made from GM corn, though since there is no labeling required, there is no way to know for sure! Best bet, steer clear of the HFCS in breads. Instead, toast up some of that French bread: dip it in spaghetti sauce, sprinkle it with cinnamon and sugar, or just eat it plain. It tastes so good, not being loaded with preservatives.

11. *Frozen fruit.* Great for little fingers. Camouflages as a frozen treat and is also good for a topping on white yogurt.

12. *Smoothies.* You know how to make them, and if you've done

them for breakfast, you should have made enough for two servings and kept one stored in your fridge or your freezer. Toss in a
few ice cubes to freshen it up and you've got a great after-school
snack!

13. *Toast.* It's not just for breakfast anymore. Top it with a piece
of chemical-free cheese, or some jelly or some cinnamon (obviously this one is a fave of the little culinary wonders in our house).

14. *Hard-boiled eggs.* Another great cook-once, eat-twice solution. Boil them up for breakfast and save one in the fridge for
later. Obviously, not for kids like Tory, but a great snack for little
hands.

I suspect that you are getting the hang of this. Just think like your
grandmother does or did. She would be so proud of you. And put your
kids to work. You don't have time to do everything, do you? And aren't
they under your feet anyway? Ten little fingers can do a lot with seven
little Tupperware pots! It's a great project for the "witching hour."

Seven Dinners

1. *Mini pizza pies.* The amazing part about these is that they
actually take less time to make than it takes to cook a frozen pizza
that you've just pulled out of the freezer—and believe me, I used
the frozen kind for years! Top English muffins with spaghetti
sauce, rBGH-free cheese (or rice cheese/almond cheese/Parme-
san: you decide what works). Add your choice of toppings: spinach?
tomatoes? salami? sausage? bacon? Get the kids involved, buffet-
line style. It will keep them preoccupied rather than picking
on each other or fighting, while you heat the oven to about 400
degrees. They make their own pies—grating cheese is a favorite
pastime in our house, as is ladling on the sauce, dropping on
the toppings, and so on. Mine usually want both halves of the
English muffin, but that is obviously dependent on the age and

appetite of the kid. Throw them in the oven for about five minutes. Done.

2. *Quesadillas.* Think of tortillas as grilled-cheese sandwiches with a boost. Choose the cheese that works for you, throw in some spinach, an avocado or guacamole if you can afford to (I try to spring for an avocado once a week since they tend to be expensive), tomatoes, and maybe some chicken from last night's dinner (remember: cook once, eat twice) or some of that leftover ground turkey that you used on the rice and beans. Put it into a giant frying pan drizzled with olive oil. Remember to think like the French moms do: they don't use a pan spray that is made from GM soy, since they don't want to feed that soy to their livestock and they don't want that spray on their food!

3. *Rice and beans.* Grab some quick-cook rice, put it into a pot with some water, bring to a boil, reduce the heat, and simmer. Drizzle olive oil into a frying pan and add some ground meat (we opt for ground turkey) and brown it (add water if necessary to keep it from sticking and creating more work at cleanup). Cover with a lid. Put some beans into a pan, and heat them up. Mix it all together when the rice is cooked, top with guacamole, salsa, and chopped-up avocado if you can afford it. If you like, add onions, tomatoes, cheese, or whatever your kid will tolerate. And have them help chop. It gets them out from underfoot and helps to prevent the fights that inevitably seem to break out around dinnertime!

4. *French night.* Bring a pot of water to boil, add some olive oil (it's a healthy source of fat and it prevents the noodles from sticking). Throw in a bag of noodles when the water has boiled, and eight minutes later, drain. Have one of your kids start drizzling olive oil (or if you're still breaking the fluorescent orange powder addiction, then use only 80 percent of the pack), and have another grate some rBGH-free cheese. Have another kid cut whole bananas into four chunks (the skin stays on to avoid the "gross brown bruises"). The third kid (or you!) gets out carrot sticks while

you grab that loaf of fresh bread from the grocery store bakery and put the rest of the cheese out on a plate on the table. This is the night that you decide to go meat-free, which I learned from Deborah Garcia can be your contribution to help reduce global warming, since the production of meat, through the extensive livestock industry, has now been shown to play a role in global warming (source: Environmental Working Group).

5. *Chicken breast night.* I love this one as it always qualifies for a "cook it once, eat it twice." Serve up the Grammy Nuggets on page 249 along with tomato wraps (sliced up tomatoes or the little cherry ones, wrapped in spinach leaves). If your kid freaks about the tomato and spinach combo, tell him to at least make one. Chances are he'll have so much fun wrapping up the tomatoes that his curiosity will be piqued over the taste. Serve with noodles drizzled with olive oil (think French moms).

6. *Pop's pork chops.* These work along the same lines as Grammy's nuggets. Throw a few pork chops in a frying pan with some olive oil and water (frozen chops are fine, though they will take longer). Then get your kids to add some salt, pepper, and garlic, put on the lid, and steam away, keeping an eye on the water, as you may need to add some. Grab the rice that is left over from rice and beans night, add a little more water to it and steam it back up. Maybe some carrot sticks? Some frozen peas? Or an apple sliced into eight pieces with that new slicer?

7. *Ground beef or ground turkey.* You can either go Mexican or make meatballs. Same rules apply as they did to the chicken and pork chops. If it's frozen, fine, though it will take longer and have to be Mexican, but add it to the frying pan with olive oil and water (are you starting to get the hang of this?) and let your kids do the spicing, cover and steam, keeping an eye on the water level (can you tell that I've burned some meat in my lifetime?). If you have rice and beans left over, mix all three up. If you have some tortillas lying around, layer all three into them and top with some

healthy cheese, salsa, or guacamole. Add an onion, some tomato, or some spinach.

If the meat is thawed out, then crack an egg into it (if your kid has no egg allergies), add some spices, then mold it into meatballs and add to the skillet that already has olive oil and water in it. While you're at it, grab the noodles that you served last night out of the fridge, reheat with some water in a pan, and get your five-year-old spiraling that rBGH-free cheese. Serve it up with the fresh bread from the bakery section (provided your husband hasn't already demolished it) and you are good to go.

Teach Your Children Well

So now you've got some ideas for how to take some baby steps in your kitchen, but maybe at this point you're wondering whether I—or my kids—are from another planet. "Maybe that worked with *her* kids," you may be thinking, "but it sure as heck won't work with mine!"

But I want to assure you that the process that the six of us went through was full of ups and downs, with its fair share of tantrums, half-eaten meals, and despair. Colin didn't want to give up his three glasses of milk a night *or* his blue yogurt. Lexy fought like a demon for her hot lunches. John was hugely attached to his three slices of pizza on pizza day. The only reason Tory didn't make a fuss was that she was not quite one when we started this whole journey, so she never knew any other way.

What I have learned is that we parents are often all too prone to make the same mistakes the food industry has made. They tried to dumb us down—is cooking a bag of noodles any more time-consuming or difficult than cooking noodles out of a blue box?—and we often inadvertently dumb down our kids, failing to give them credit for being able to think, draw conclusions, and solve problems. They tried to hide the true content of their "convenience" foods and sugary cereals—and we often try to slip one over on our kids, failing to disclose our actions and intentions as well.

So if you have made it this far along and are still concerned about what your kids are eating, honor their brains and fully disclose what you are doing and why. Explain to your children that chemicals can hurt their tummies, their insides, their heads. Tell them you love them too much to give them food that you now understand may be bad for them. Find an age-appropriate and non-scary way to help them picture what the chemicals might do and help them visualize what healthy foods can do. Help them discover how those "fake foods" affect them.

"Let's see how much better you feel when you don't have those things swimming around inside of you!" I used to say to Colin, or Lexy, or John. "Let's notice how you act on the days when you eat that hot lunch. Let's see how your tummy feels, or your head. Wow, there's an angry face—do you think it has anything to do with what you had for lunch today? Let's play detective—let me know if your poops ever get too runny. Kind of gross, sure, but Mommy is trying to help you to feel better, so you have to be Mommy's teacher! Let's see if we can figure out which kinds of foods help you act the best."

Here are some useful "teaching" phrases that you might try with your kids:

- "If you choose to eat this now, let's see how you feel and act later."
- "Did that food make you feel grouchy? Hyper? Sad? Maybe next time you eat it, you can pay attention and then I'll ask you how you feel."
- "Did that food give you a headache? Itchy skin? Watery eyes? You're not sure? Okay, the next time you eat it, let's both pay attention and see what happens."
- "Honey, I've noticed that when you drink blue juice you sometimes get hyper—have you noticed that? What happens when you get hyper? Will you get in trouble for bad behavior? What do teachers do when they see a hyper kid? What do I do when you are

like that? What else usually happens? Do you get hurt? Do you
fight with your brother or sister? How does that make you feel?"

If you are weaning your kids from something that has bad effects on
them, either because they're allergic or because they're responding to the
chemicals, be prepared for a long, slow process. When we were weaning
Colin from his three glasses of milk a night, I started by giving him only
two glasses. He had to have water for the last glass.

The next step was to cut back to two partial glasses—since they were
given in sippy cups, he couldn't tell that the glasses were less full. Then
we made it one, and finally, none.

Along the way, I talked him through it. "Colin, you know how your
armpits get red and sore and really hurt? That is a reaction to all the milk
you're drinking, so we need to try to get you to drink less milk, so your
armpits don't get sore. Do you want sore armpits?"

"No, Mommy, but I want more milk!"

"Well, you can have *some* milk. Tonight, you can have two glasses."

"But I want three!"

"Sorry, Colin. Tonight, it's two."

And then if there was a tantrum, there was. (My final response was always, "You know, you could always have *none!*") I wouldn't let my kid go
into the deep end of the pool by himself, or cross a busy street alone, or
eat three big pieces of birthday cake. If saying no to those things provoked a tantrum—and all of us have been there!—I'd just have been prepared to ride it out. The milk really wasn't any different.

I also used to involve my kids in making healthy choices. I showed
them how to read labels and how to find foods in the grocery store, and
I asked for their help in choosing chemical-free foods (the ones without
those long words in the labels) and avoiding the ones loaded with chemicals (the ones with the "#" in the label, or the ones that list ingredients
we can't pronounce much less spell). It took some time, for sure, but I
was investing in them. And ultimately, it saved time down the road, as I
taught my kids to be their own little anti-chemical crusaders.

If you teach your kids to make their own smart choices, then the battleground will fade away. They will be empowered smart kids that you will be so proud of.

This Is a Carrot

One of the great things about taking your first baby step toward healthier eating is that you just feel so good about it. You are so proud of doing something to help your family, and it's so empowering to take any action at all. The good feelings you get motivate you to take the next step, and the next one, and the next. The good responses you eventually get from your kids—and from your own renewed health—are wonderfully reinforcing as well.

One of my favorite rewards in this process came, once again, from Colin. Now, when we started this whole process in the winter of 2006, Colin literally freaked out at the very sight of a vegetable. I'm not exaggerating: if he so much as saw a carrot sitting on his plate, he'd lose it. The deal we had to make with him, when we started switching our diets, was that the carrot would stay *on the table,* in front of his plate, not on it.

Eventually—maybe six or seven months later—Colin agreed that the dreaded carrot could rest upon his sacred plate. Progress!

Three or four months after that, we got him to try a "mouse bite."

"Yuck! I *hate* it!" he'd always say—but at least, after a while, he'd swallow. Then we asked, "Is this a big mouse or a little one?"

Well, last night at dinner, the very day I'd been typing up the notes for this chapter, I saw Colin pick up an entire carrot and take a big bite out of the end. He chewed it thoughtfully, then pulled the half-bitten stick out of his mouth.

"You know, Mom," he said casually, as though he'd just noticed something barely worth mentioning, "I sorta like carrots."

I felt as though someone had just given me the Mother's Medal of

Honor. And when your kids are eating your new, healthy, junk-free diet, so will you.

Chances are that not only are you a better cook than I am, but that you are also way ahead of where I was when I started this. So, go for it! If it helps to keep in mind the words of Christopher Robin to Winnie-the-Pooh, *"Promise me you'll always remember: You're braver than you believe, and stronger than you seem, and smarter than you think."* And when your Medal of Honor day comes, you have to let me know!

ACKNOWLEDGMENTS

This book, written in memory of Colette Chuda and Emily Vonder Meulen, reflects the work of several remarkable lives.

My agent, Carrie Cook, had the vision to see the potential for a book that far exceeded anything that I could have hoped for. She is compassionate, brilliant, savvy, and kind. Her friendship, strength, and wisdom have been gifts to me and my family.

Broadway Books editor in chief, Stacy Creamer, directed every detail and nuance with a heartfelt depth of insight, talent, and experience that I find awe-inspiring. I am extremely honored by her work on this book, as I consider her one of the most talented editors in the publishing world. Her candor, sense of humor, and knowledge were critical in the process. Her team, including Ann Campbell, is an incredible inspiration.

Rachel Kranz, my coauthor, brought the book to a level that I never would have accomplished alone. Rachel challenged me in ways that I could not have imagined, and her intelligence is unrivaled. I am extremely grateful for her courage, honesty, and encouragement. I am so proud to have Rachel as a friend and to have worked with her experienced agent, Janis Vallely.

To Erin Brockovich, Michael Pollan, and Mehmet Oz, it is with sincere gratitude that I thank you for your kindness and words of encouragement, as they often came at times when our family needed them most.

To Nell Newman and Bobby Kennedy, thank you for listening, for responding, and for pushing me forward.

To Sally Shepherd, from "behind the scenes," you blew wind into my sails in times of need, for which I can't thank you enough.

To Drs. Kenneth Bock, David Ludwig, and Joel Fuhrman, thank you for believing in my work. You are gifts to an entire generation of children, and I will be forever indebted to you for your courageous efforts in pursuing this truth.

To Michael Hansen, Chuck Benbrook, Deborah Koons Garcia, Nancy Chuda, John Reganold, Rick North, and Sonya Lunder, thank you for your pioneering work and for taking the time to teach me the science behind our food supply.

To Erik Bruun Bindslev, your support and friendship are treasured gifts, for which I will be forever grateful. And to Rice University's Jones's Graduate School's associate professor Doug Schuler, your ethics course profoundly changed how I viewed the world.

To my mom, for her compassion and for teaching me to look at the world through a wide-angle lens; to my dad, who taught me to always give 110 percent, and to my beautiful nieces, nephews, and godchildren and the millions that you represent—including Roman, Danny, and Kevin—the value of your lives is immeasurable.

To Allison Doering, Lizzie Parks, and my husband's family, I would not have survived without your love and support.

To my sporty friends in Boulder, thank you for your friendship, wit and wisdom and the constant reminder that the pursuit of a passion is not without sacrifice, hard work, and a healthy dose of compulsion!

To my children—Lexy, Colin, John, and Tory—you are my inspiration to make the world a better place, and I am so proud of you. You flood my heart with courage, love, and hope.

To my husband, Jeff, there are not words to convey the depth of emotion that I have for you. Your kindness and wisdom nourish me and your unconditional love makes me whole. You are the most remarkable person I know.

To those who have gone before me and those who will follow, it is with inspired hope and profound gratitude that I thank you for the work that you have done and continue to do for the health of our children.

APPENDIX: ORGANIC 101

Health Benefits

A recent study into organic food found that it appears to:
- Strengthen your immune system
- Improve sleeping habits
- Cut the risk of cancers
- Reduce the risks of heart disease
- Reduce a child's exposure to hidden allergens
- Promote weight loss

As you can imagine, the junk food industry's un-organic response to this groundswell of healthy food choices is to highlight industry-funded research that suggests that eating organic food is no more than a lifestyle choice. Thankfully, an insightful four-year, $25 million European study found that:

- Animals fed an organic diet were slimmer (yes, skinnier!) than their un-organic-fed counterparts because fat cells appear to trap and store the heavy pesticide residues found in un-organic produce.
- Organics appear to promote weight loss by reducing your exposure to chemical pesticides that bind to fat and once absorbed may stay in the body for a lifetime (over 350 chemicals can accumulate in our body fat!).
- Organic fruit and vegetables contain up to 40 percent more antioxidants.
- Milk from organic herds contained up to 90 percent more antioxidants.
- Organic food also had higher levels of beneficial minerals such as iron and zinc, critical minerals in the development of a child's brain.

Additionally, according to the Center for Food Safety, un-organic crops like corn and soy that have been genetically engineered to be more profitable now contain chemical toxins in their seeds, which may be why these crops are banned in Europe, Australia, Japan, Russia, and almost forty developed countries around the world. They may also contain hidden allergens that might be contributing to the allergy epidemic.

So What Does "Organic" Mean? And What About "All Natural"?

Because the United States lags behind other developed countries when it comes to food safety, understanding label claims can often be a challenge for even the savviest shopper.

The term "organic" refers to foods grown and processed without chemical toxins, artificial ingredients, chemical preservatives, or ionizing radiation. The guidelines for organic foods were established on October 21, 2002, by the U.S. Department of Agriculture. To use these terms, producers must pay additional fees and follow strict guidelines and regulations:

- 100% Organic—All ingredients are organic.
- Organic—95 percent or more of the total ingredients are organic.
- Made with Organic Ingredients—At least 70 percent of the ingredients are organic.

For the savviest of label readers, the following are the legal guidelines established by the U.S. Department of Agriculture for organics:

Organic Fruits and Vegetables
Must be grown without the use of:
- synthetically created chemical pesticides
- synthetically created chemical fertilizers
- sewage sludge
- genetic engineering that appears to introduce novel proteins, allergens, viruses, and toxins into crops
- irradiation (a type of chemotherapy for produce)

Organic Beef and Chicken
- Fed only 100 percent organic feed, are not the offspring of cloned animals, and have never been administered growth hormones or antibiotics. In addition, their meat must never be irradiated.

- Natural (or All Natural) meat or poultry products contain no artificial ingredients and are minimally processed. They are not necessarily organic.

- "No hormones administered" or "no antibiotics added" is sometimes seen on labels, but it can only appear if the producer can document the absence of hormone or antibiotic administration.

- Free-range or free-roaming poultry have access to the outdoors without a minimum time. They are not necessarily organic.

- Cage-free poultry means nothing as most chickens are kept indoors (but cage-free) if they are grown for meat.

Organic Milk

Comes from animals that were fed 100 percent organic feed and were not given antibiotics, prophylactic drugs, or genetically engineered and synthetically created growth hormones (such as rBGH) for at least the last year.

RBGH (recombinant bovine growth hormone) is a genetically engineered, synthetic chemical protein hormone vaccinated into cows to artificially boost their milk production. Like aspartame and other chemicals, rBGH is not found in foods in Europe, Canada, Asia, and around the world.

Organic Eggs

- Produced by hens that are fed 100 percent organic feed and have never been given growth hormones or antibiotics.

- Cage-free eggs are produced by hens that are not confined in cages. The hens might not have access to the outdoors, though, and are not necessarily organic.

Organic Seafood

The USDA currently has no guidelines set for seafood; however, farm-raised fish is often caged underwater and treated with pesticides to prevent the spread of disease.

Organic Bread

Cereal and grain crops are regularly sprayed with pesticides that collect in the grain's outer layers, raising concerns about chemical residues in un-organic bread, cakes, and cookies.

Other Terms

The following terms are often found on packaged products and can be confusing to consumers:

Natural is often a misnomer. There are no true guidelines for this term when used on a packaged product, although it is used frequently and often assumed to mean organic or healthier.

Gourmet is another misleading term that leads consumers to believe that they are purchasing a product made with finer ingredients, when in reality there are no established guidelines or regulations.

The Dirty Dozen

According to the Environmental Working Group, "The Dirty Dozen" is a list of twelve fruits and vegetables that contain the highest levels of chemical and pesticide residues. In order to avoid this pesticide-drenched produce, you may want to "opt out" of the items on this list or consider their organic substitutes if your budget allows:

- Peaches
- Apples
- Sweet bell peppers
- Celery
- Nectarines
- Strawberries
- Cherries
- Lettuce
- Imported grapes
- Pears
- Spinach
- Potatoes

RESOURCES

Grocery Store Resources

Brands to Look for in the Grocery Store

These are suggestions, not a complete list. And always, *always* check the label, as food manufacturers can change their ingredient list at any time!

GMO-free Grocery Store Brands
Safeway Organics
Publix Green Wise products
Kroger Naturally Preferred products
Trader Joe's

Dairy
Safeway Organics
Horizon Organic
Stonyfield Farm Organic
Organic Valley Dairy
Ben & Jerry's Ice Cream
Tillamook Cheese

Eggs
Organic Valley
Nest Fresh Organics
Land O'Lakes Organics

Baby Food and Infant Formula
Gerber Products
Earth's Best
Baby's Only
Horizon Organic
Safeway Organics

Fast and Easy: Prepackaged Boxes and Bags

Ketchups, Sauces, Condiments, and Salad Dressing
Annie's
Muir Glen
Marantha Nut Butters
Safeway Organics
Seeds of Change
Amy's Kitchen
Newman's Own Organic and Newman's Own (except salad dressing)
Health Valley Organic
Nature's Path Organics
Barbara's Organic
Hain Pure Foods
Santa Cruz Organic
Rudi's Own Organics
Nogurt

Snack Bars
Clif Bars
Luna Bars
Odwalla
Fruta Bu

Boxes to Bake With
Arrowhead Mills (organic)
Bob's Red Mill (organic)
Eden Organics

Cereal
EnviroKidz
Nature's Path

Cascadian Farms (Clifford Crunch is a favorite in our house!)
Barbara's Organic
Health Valley Organic

Candy and Chocolate
Newman's Own
Ghirardelli Chocolate
Yummy Earth
St. Claire Organic
Pure Fun
Jelly Belly

Juices
Santa Cruz Organic
Knudsen Organic
Eden Organics
Cascadian Farms
Odwalla
NUI Water

Web Resources

AllergyKids
www.AllergyKids.com

Allergy Elimination Techniques
www.naet.com

Alliance for Biointegrity
www.biointegrity.org

Autism Speaks
www.autismspeaks.org

Breast Cancer Fund
www.pureprevention.org

Cancer Prevention Coalition
www.preventcancer.com

Center for Food Safety
www.centerforfoodsafety.org

Chemical Free Kids
www.chemicalfreekids.com

Council on Foreign Relations
www.cfr.org

Defeat Autism Now: A Project of the Autism Research Institute
www.autism.com/dan/

Environmental Health News
www.environmentalhealthnews.org

Environmental Working Group
www.ewg.org

Environmental Working Group's Food News
http://foodnews.org/

Feingold Association
www.feingold.org

Food and Behavior Research
www.lobbywatch.org

Food and Water Watch
www.foodandwaterwatch.org

Food Matters
www.foodmatters.com

Food Navigator
www.foodnavigator.com

Grass Fed Meats
www.texasgrassfedbeef.com

Healthy Child Healthy World
www.healthychild.org

Institute for Responsible Technology
www.seedsofdeception.com

International Food Ingredients: Food Colors and the Law
www.ifi-online.com/Tmpl_Article.asp?ContentID=272&ContentType=3

National Eating Disorders Association
www.nationaleatingdisorders.org

Newman's Own Organics
www.newmansownorganics.com

Open Secrets
www.opensecrets.org

Oregon Physicians for Social Responsibility
www.oregonpsr.org

The Organic and Non-GMO Report
www.non-gmoreport.com

The Organic Center
www.organic-center.org

Organic Consumers Association
www.organicconsumers.org

The Ramazzini Foundation: Portal on the Research and
Prevention of Cancer
www.ramazzini.it

Rodale Institute
www.rodaleinstitute.org

The Soil Association
www.soilassociation.org

Source Watch
www.sourcewatch.org

Soy Online Service
www.soyonlineservice.co.nz

Take Part
www.takepart.com/foodinc

Your Milk on Drugs
www.yourmilkondrugs.com

Books

I know it's hard for busy people to work more reading into their schedule. So I've listed these books in their order of importance to me. If you don't know where to start, you might begin at the beginning of the list.

Kenneth Bock, MD. *Healing the New Childhood Epidemics: Autism, ADHD, Asthma and Allergies.* Random House, 2007.

Marc Schapiro. *Exposed: The Toxic Chemistry of Everyday Products and What's at Stake for American Power.* Chelsea Green Publishing, 2007.

Nell Newman, with Joseph D'Agnese. *The Newman's Own Organics Guide to a Good Life: Simple Measures That Benefit You and the Place You Live.* Villard Books/Random House, 2003.

Ann Cooper and Lisa M. Holmes. *Lunch Lessons: Changing the Way We Feed Our Children.* HarperCollins, 2006.

David Zinczenko and Matt Goulding. *Eat This Not That: Thousands of Simple Food Swaps That Can Save You 10, 20, 30 Pounds—or More!* Rodale Press, December 2007.

T. Colin Campbell and Thomas M. Campbell II. *The China Study: The Most Comprehensive Study of Nutrition Ever Conducted and the Startling Implications for Diet, Weight Loss and Long-term Health.* Benbella Books, 2006.

Carol Simontacchi. *The Crazy Makers: How the Food Industry Is Destroying Our Brains and Harming Our Children.* Penguin Books, 2000.

Eric Schlosser and Charles Wilson. *Chew on This.* Houghton Mifflin, 2006.

Andrew Kimbrell. *Your Right to Know: Genetic Engineering and the Secret Changes in Your Food.* Earth Aware Editions, 2007.

Jeffrey M. Smith. *Genetic Roulette, The Documented Health Risks of Genetically Engineered Foods.* Yes! Books, 2007.

———. *Seeds of Deception: Exposing Industry and Government Lies About the Safety of the Genetically Engineered Foods You're Eating.* Yes! Books, 2003.

Michael Pollan. *In Defense of Food: An Eater's Manifesto.* Penguin Press, 2008.

———. *The Omnivore's Dilemma.* Penguin Books, 2006.

Russell L. Blaylock. *Excitotoxins: The Taste That Kills.* Health Press, 1996.

Randall Fitzgerald. *The Hundred Year Life: How to Protect Yourself from the Chemicals That Are Destroying Your Health.* Plume, 2007.

Thomas R. Pawlick. *The End of Food: How the Food Industry Is Destroying Our Food Supply—And What We Can Do About It.* Barricade Books, 2006.

Kim Barnouin and Rory Freedman. *Skinny Bitch.* Running Press, 2005.

Joseph Mercola and Kendra Degen Pearsall. *Sweet Deception: Why Splenda, NutraSweet, and the FDA May Be Hazardous to Your Health.* Nelson Books, 2006.

Sally Fallon. *Nourishing Traditions: The Cookbook That Challenges Politically Correct Nutrition and the Diet Dictocrats.* New Trends Publishing, 1999.

Kaayla Daniel. *The Whole Soy Story: The Dark Side of America's Favorite Health Food.* New Trends Publishing, 2005.

Mehmet Oz and Michael F. Roizen. *YOU: The Owner's Manual, Updated and Expanded Edition: An Insider's Guide to the Body That Will Make You Healthier and Younger.* HarperCollins Living, updated 2008.

Jessica Seinfeld. *Deceptively Delicious: Simple Secrets to Get Your Kids Eating Good Food.* HarperCollins, 2007.

Films

Again, I've listed these films in what I consider priority order. So if you're looking to prioritize, just start at the beginning of the list.

The Future of Food
A film by Deborah Koons Garcia
Lily Films
P.O. Box 895
Mill Valley, CA 94942
Tel: (800) 981-7870
E-mail: customerservice@futureoffoodstore.com
http://www.thefutureoffood.com/involved.htm

Food, Inc.
Participant Media LLC
Tel: (866) 9-TAKEPART
E-mail: feedback@takepart.com
http://www.takepart.com/foodinc
http://www.participantmedia.com/films/Coming+Soon/517/FoodInc

King Corn
A feature documentary by Mosaic Films Incorporated
Tel: (503) 863-7270
http://www.kingcorn.net

Generation Rx
A film by Kevin P. Miller and Common Radius Films
Common Radius Films
240-196 West Third Ave.
Vancouver, BC V5Y 1E9
Tel: (604) 639-3337
Fax: (604) 876-6649
E-mail: info@commonradius.com
http://www.generationrxfilm.com

The World According to Monsanto: A Documentary That Americans Won't Ever See
A film by Marie-Monique Robin
Mongrel Media
1028 Queen Street West
Toronto, ON M6J 1H6
Tel: (416) 516-9775
Fax: (416) 516-0651
E-mail: info@mongrelmedia.com
http://www.mongrelmedia.com

The Corporation
By Mark Achbar, Jennifer Abbott, and Joel Bakan
http://www.thecorporation.com

Michael Clayton
Smoke House Pictures
4000 Warner Blvd., Bldg. 15
Burbank, CA 91522
Tel: (818) 954-4840
Fax: (818) 954-4860
http://www.clooneystudio.com/michaelclayton.html

NOTES

Introduction: A Reluctant Crusader

one out of every seventeen children:

2   www.foodallergy.org, Food Allergy and Anaphylaxis Network (FAAN) Web site, accessed January 2006.

one out of every three U.S. kids:

2   Kenneth Bock, *Healing the New Childhood Epidemics: Autism, ADHD, Asthma and Allergies* (Random House, 2007).

peanut allergies:

2   Scott Sicherer, Anne Munoz-Furlong, and Hugh A. Sampson, "Prevalence of Peanut and Tree Nut Allergy in the United States Determined by Means of a Random Digit Dial Telephone Survey: A 5-Year Follow-up Study," *Journal of Allergy and Clinical Immunology* 112, no. 6 (2003): 1203–7.

Chapter 1. Baby Steps

proteins in eight foods:

9   www.aaaai.org, American Academy of Allergy, Asthma and Immunology Web site, accessed January 2006.

the official statistic:

14   Lester M. Crawford, Consumer Federation of America, Washington, D.C., Public Speeches, April 22, 2002, http://www.fda.gov/oc/speeches/2002.html.

"Over the last 20 years":

14   Robert A. Wood, with Joe Kraynak, *Food Allergies for Dummies* (Wiley
      Publishing, 2007), p. 38.

"I've been treating children":

15   A. Wesley Burks, "'Don't Feed Her That!' Diagnosing and Managing
      Pediatric Food Allergy," *Pediatric Basics,* no. 115 (2006).

peanut allergies among children:

15   Scott Sicherer, Anne Munoz-Furlong, and Hugh A. Sampson, "Preva-
      lence of Peanut and Tree Nut Allergy in the United States Determined
      by Means of a Random Digit Dial Telephone Survey: A 5-Year Follow-up
      Study," *Journal of Allergy and Clinical Immunology* 112, no. 6 (2003):
      1203–7.

"Estimates have been":

15   Burks, "'Don't Feed Her That!'"

a 265 percent increase:

16   Ibid.; Karen Ann Cullotta, "Researchers Put a Microscope on Food Al-
      lergies," *New York Times,* December 9, 2008, http://www.nytimes.com/
      2008/12/09/health/09allergies.html?em =&pagewanted=print; Sam Roe,
      "Children at Risk in Food Roulette: Mislabeling, lax oversight threatens
      people with allergies," *Chicago Tribune,* November 21, 2008, http:
      //www.chicagotribune.com/features/lifestyle/health/chi-081120-
      allergens-tribune-investigation,0,506031.story; Amy M. Branum and
      Susan L. Lukacs, "Food Allergy Among U.S. Children: Trends in Preva-
      lence and Hospitalizations," NCHS Data Brief no. 10, October 2008,
      http://www.cdc.gov/nchs/data/databriefs/db10.pdf; Centers for Disease
      Control, "CDC Study Finds 3 Million U.S. Children Have Food or Di-
      gestive Allergies," October 22, 2008, http://www.cdc.gov/media/pressrel/
      2008/r081022.htm.

number of children with seasonal allergies:

16   Claudia Kalb, "Medicine: Fear and Allergies in the Lunchroom,"
      Newsweek, November 5, 2007.

"The severity of those allergies":

16   Ibid.

"There are no studies":
16   Burks, "'Don't Feed Her That!'"

a study in Great Britain:
17   Peter W. Bennett, Leonard M. McEwen, Helen C. McEwen, and Eunice L. Rose, "The Shipley Project: Treating Food Allergy to Prevent Criminal Behavior in Community Setting," *Journal of Nutritional and Environmental Medicine* 8 (1998): 77–83; Carol Simontacchi, *The Crazy Makers: How the Food Industry Is Destroying Our Brains and Harming Our Children* (Penguin Books, 2000), p. 168.

Scientists now believe:
18   Richard Coico, Geoffrey Sunshine, and Eli Benjamini, *Immunology: A Short Course* (Wiley-Liss, 2003).

symptoms may also combine:
19   Cleveland Clinic Center for Consumer Health Information, http://www.clevelandclinic.org/health.

Common Symptoms of Food Allergy:
20   http:www.webmd.com and http:www.clevelandclinic.org/health; Kenneth Bock, MD, personal communication, April 30, 2008.

Common Symptoms of Food Sensitivity:
20   Kenneth Bock, MD, personal communication, April 30, 2008.

number of deaths caused by asthma:
21   Asthma and Allergy Foundation of America, www.aafa.org, accessed July 2008; *Asthma Facts and Figures,* http://www.aafa.org/display.cfm?id=8&sub=42; "New Asthma Estimates: Tracking Prevalence, Health Care and Mortality," National Center for Health Statistics, Centers for Disease Control, 2001, http://www.cdc.gov/nchs/pressroom/01facts/asthma.htm.

asthma causes 40,000 U.S. residents:
21   Ibid.

"asthma and allergies strike 1 in 4":
21   Ibid.

"Reliable asthma studies":
22   Wood, *Food Allergies for Dummies,* p. 38.

doctors prescribe antihistamines:
23   D. D. Metcalfe, D. Baram, and Y. A. Mekori, "Mast Cells," *Physiological Reviews* 77, no. 4 (October 1977): 1033–79. PubMed Identifier 9354811, http://www.ncbi.nlm.nih.gov/pubmed/9354811.

linked mast cells:
23   Theoharis C. Theoharides, "Mast Cells and Pancreatic Cancer," *New England Journal of Medicine* 358, no. 17 (April 24, 2008): 1860–61.

contributes to other disorders:
23   M. G. Borrello, D. Degl'innocenti, and M. A. Pierotti, "Inflammation and Cancer: The Oncogene-driven Connection," PubMed Identifier 18502035, http://www.ncbi.nlm.nih.gov/pubmed/18502035?ordinalpos=9&itool= EntrezSystem2.PEntrez.Pubmed.Pubmed_ResultsPanel.Pubmed_ RVDocSum.

Allergies of all types:
23   Sean Flynn, "What You Can Do About Food Allergies," *Parade,* April 29, 2007, http://www.parade.com/articles/editions/2007/edition_04-29-2007/ Food_Allergies: " 'Food allergies have exploded in recent decades . . . the rise is also real, dramatic and documented. We're basically looking at what may be a public-health crisis, and we have to find ways to deal with it,' says Dr. Scott H. Sicherer, a researcher at the Jaffe Food Allergy Institute at Mount Sinai School of Medicine in New York City."

The potential dangers:
24   Bock, *Healing the New Childhood Epidemics.*

prevalence of food sensitivity:
26   H. M. Anthony et al., "Food Intolerance," *The Lancet* 344 (July 9, 1994): 136–37.

"Both categories have been exploding":
27   Dr. Kenneth Bock, personal communication, April 30, 2008.

children may develop food sensitivities:

28   D. McCann et al., "Food Additives and Hyperactive Behaviour in 3-year-old and 8/9-year-old Children in the Community: A Randomised, Double-blinded, Placebo-controlled Trial," *The Lancet* 370, no. 9598 (November 3, 2007).

Even when your kid is too young:

29   Bock, *Healing the New Childhood Epidemics.*

Chapter 2. Becoming the Allergy Detective

"No one really knows":

38   Robert Wood, "Food Allergies for Dummies," http://drrobertwood.com/food-allergy-epidemic.shtml, accessed July 23, 2008.

"The human race hasn't changed":

39   Claudia Kalb, "Medicine: Fear and Allergies in the Lunchroom," *Newsweek*, November 5, 2007.

environmental pollution:

39   Ibid.

increased levels of environmental toxins:

39   Dr. Kenneth Bock, personal communication, April 30, 2008.

"An allergic reaction":

40   Ibid.

The kids from the bigger families:

40   David P. Strachan, "Hay Fever, Hygiene, and Household Size," *British Medical Journal* 299 (1989): 1259–60.

Since 1989, scientists:

40   F. Guarner et al., "Mechanisms of Disease: The Hygiene Hypothesis Revisited," *Nature Clinical Practice Gastroenterology & Hepatology* 3 (2006): 275–84.

More recent research:

41   Kalb, "Medicine: Fear and Allergies in the Lunchroom."

Dr. Wood adds that:

41 Robert A. Wood, with Joe Kraynak, *Food Allergies for Dummies* (Wiley Publishing, 2007), pp. 38–39.

"many researchers say":

41 Kenneth Bock, *Healing the New Childhood Epidemics: Autism, ADHD, Asthma and Allergies* (Random House, 2007).

"some of the highest rates":

43 Wood, "Food Allergies for Dummies."

switching from natural to processed:

44 Joel Fuhrman, MD, personal communication, May 6, 2008.

the global incidence of childhood allergies:

45 Konrad Rydzynskia and Cezary Palczynski, "Toxicology in the New Century, Opportunities and Challenges," International Study of Asthma and Allergies in Children, *Proceedings of the 5th Congress of Toxicology in Developing Countries* 198, nos. 1–3 (May 20, 2004): 75–82.

20 million Americans:

45 *Allergy and Asthma Advocate* (Winter 2006), http://www.aaaai.org/patients/advocate/2006/winter/winter06.pdf: "Asthma is a chronic disease that affects approximately 20 million Americans, and is responsible for nearly 5,000 deaths a year. In addition, there are nearly 2 million asthma-related visits to the emergency department each year."

some one in eight:

45 Centers for Disease Control and Prevention, March 2005, http://www.cdc.gov/asthma/children.htm.

"Asthma is an allergy":

45 Joel Fuhrman, MD, personal communication, May 6, 2008.

"a diverse array":

46 David Ludwig, MD, personal communication, May 6, 2008.

"Consuming a highly processed":

47 Ibid.

the ACAAI's own Web site:

56   Center for Science in the Public Interest, *Integrity in Science Database,*
      http://cspinet.org/integrity. "American College of Allergy, Asthma, and
      Immunology": "[A]n organization of allergists-immunologists and related
      health care professionals dedicated to quality patient care through
      research, advocacy and professional and public education. Its website
      is sponsored by an educational grant from Dura Pharmaceuticals.
      (http://www.allergy.mcg.edu/About.html, accessed February 24, 2003)."

The first project ran:

57   "Educate the Educator," National Peanut Funding Database, supported
      by the Peanut Foundation, Peanut Foundation Funding, $14,000,
      Agency/Department: Virginia Tech, April 1999–March 2000, http://
      apps.caes.uga.edu/Peanuts/results.cfm, accessed July 8, 2008.

"increase awareness of food allergy":

57   Food Allergy Network support of Food Allergy Education for Educators,
      National Peanut Funding Database, supported by the Peanut Founda-
      tion, Peanut Foundation Funding, $15,875, Agency/Department: Peanut
      Foundation, March 2000–April 2001, http://apps.caes.uga.edu/Peanuts/
      results.cfm, accessed July 8, 2008; Educate the Educator Program,
      National Peanut Funding Database, supported by the Peanut Founda-
      tion, Peanut Foundation Funding, $13,000, Agency/Department: Peanut
      Foundation, March 2005–March 2006, http://apps.caes.uga.edu/
      Peanuts/results.cfm, accessed July 8, 2008.

"funded by an educational grant":

57   Center for Science in the Public Interest, *Integrity in Science Database,*
      http://cspinet.org/integrity, accessed July 2008.

FAAN medical board member:

58   U.S. Patent 6835824, Peanut *allergens* and methods. Inventors: A. Wes-
      ley Burks, Jr., J. Steven Stanley, Gary A. Bannon, Gael Cockrell, Ricki
      M. Helm. Issued by the United States Patent and Trademark Office,
      December 28, 2004. Patent Storm, http://www.patentstorm.us/patents/
      6835824/description.html, accessed July 8, 2008.

In another Monsanto tie:

58   Center for Science in the Public Interest, *Integrity in Science Database,*
      http://cspinet.org/integrity, accessed July 2008.

coinventor on a new Monsanto protein:

58   U.S. Patent 7381556, Nucleic acids encoding deallergenized proteins
      and permuteins. Inventors: Murtaza F. Alibhai, James D. Astwood,
      Charles A. McWherter, Hugh A. Sampson. Assignee: Monsanto Tech-
      nology, LLC. Issued by the United States Patent and Trademark Office,
      June 3, 2008. Patent Storm, http://www.patentstorm.us/patents/7381556
      .html, accessed July 8, 2008.

committed to "meet the needs":

58   www.peanutbioscience.com/peanutgenomeinitiative.html, accessed De-
      cember 30, 2008.

cross-reactivity between the soybean and the peanut:

59   The Legume Information System, Peanut Genome Initiative Meeting
      Minutes, Renaissance Hotel, Portsmouth, Virginia, July 12, 2005,
      http://www.comparative-legumes.org:2000/forum/mvnforum/
      viewthread?thread=36, accessed July 8, 2008.

testified to the safety of MSG:

59   Executive Summary, "Analysis of Adverse Reactions to Monosodium Glu-
      tamate (MSG)," Center for Food Safety and Applied Nutrition, Food and
      Drug Administration, Department of Health and Human Services, Wash-
      ington, D.C. 20204 under FDA Contract No. 223-92-2185, Task Orders
      No. 1 and 7. Published as a supplement to the *Journal of Nutrition* 125
      (1995): 2891S–2906S, http://jn.nutrition.org/cgi/reprint/125/11/2891S
      .pdf, accessed July 8, 2008.

controversial artificial sweetener:

59   UPI Investigative Report, "NutraSweet: Questions Swirl," 1987,
      http://www.dorway.com/upipaper.txt, accessed July 8, 2008.

When I first discovered these connections:

59   Steve Charles, "Scientist Cites Ethical Imperative for Modified Crops,"
      http://www.wabash.edu/academics/chemistry/departments.cfm?pages
      _ id=2&news_ID=4499, accessed March 16, 2007.

Chapter 3. Soy Secrets

"In effect, children are used":

62   Sam Roe, "Children at Risk in Food Roulette: Mislabeling, lax oversight threatens people with allergies," *Chicago Tribune,* November 21, 2008, http://www.chicagotribune.com/features/lifestyle/health/chi-081120-allergens-tribune-investigation,0,506031.story, accessed November 22, 2008.

Angola, Malawi, Mozambique:

64   Robert Paarlberg et al., "Food Aid Import Policies in the COMESA/ASARECA Region: The Costs and Benefits of Current Policy Options," African Centre for Technology Studies, Nairobi, Kenya, 2006, http://www.acts.or.ke/pubs/monographs/pubs/rabesa_report3.pdf.

a news report about a Michigan study:

64   Venu Gangur, "Will Genetically Engineered Foods Cause Allergic Reactions? Scientists Receive EPA Grant to Find Out," http://newsroom.msu.edu/site/indexer/2864/content.htm, September 27, 2006.

fifteen soybean proteins:

65   Ricki M. Helm, A. Wesley Burks, and Eliot Herman, "Hypoallergenic Foods—Soybeans and Peanuts," *Information Systems for Biotechnology,* October 2002, http://www.isb.vt.edu/news/2002/news02.oct.html#oct0202, accessed August 1, 2008.

trypsin inhibitor:

65   Stephen R. Padgette et al., "The Composition of Glyphosate-Tolerant Soybean Seeds Is Equivalent to That of Conventional Soybeans," *Journal of Nutrition* 126, no. 4 (April 1996). In Jeffrey M. Smith, *Seeds of Deception: Exposing Industry and Government Lies About the Safety of the Genetically Engineered Foods You're Eating* (Yes! Books, 2003), p. 161.

U.K. rate of soy allergies:

66   Smith, *Seeds of Deception,* p. 160.

possible links between soy allergies:

67   Helm, Burks, and Herman, "Hypoallergenic Foods."

something called StarLink corn:

67   Luca Bucchini and Lynn R. Goldman, "StarLink Corn: A Risk Analysis,"
      Environmental Health Perspectives 110, no. 1 (January 2002): 5–13.

allergenicity of genetically modified foods:

67   Notes from the Food Biotechnology Subcommittee meeting of the Food
      Advisory Committee, August 13, 2002, Department of Health and
      Human Services, Food and Drug Administration, and Center for Food
      Safety and Applied Nutrition, http://www.fda.gov/OHRMS/DOCKETS/
      ac/02/transcripts/3886t1.doc, accessed August 1, 2008.

Sampson, currently on FAAN's medical board:

67   National Toxicology Program, Department of Health and Human Ser-
      vices, Federal Register: November 13, 2001 (vol. 66, no. 219), "Assess-
      ment of the Allergenic Potential of Genetically Modified Foods,"
      December 10–12, 2001, Chapel Hill, N.C., http://ntp.niehs.nih.gov/
      index.cfm?objectid=06F4CC5B-D093-A437-23B8AE16995A9DFE.

sponsored a joint report:

67   "Evaluation of Allergenicity of Genetically Modified Foods," Report of a
      Joint FAO/WHO Expert Consultation on Allergenicity of Foods Derived
      from Biotechnology, Food and Agriculture Organization of the United
      Nations (FAO) and the World Health Organization (WHO), Rome, Jan-
      uary 22–25, 2001, ftp://ftp.fao.org/es/esn/food/allergygm.pdf, accessed
      August 1, 2008.

expressed their concern:

68   Daniel M. Sheehan and Daniel R. Doerge, http://www.soyonlineservice
      .co.nz/downloads/nctrpti.pdf, accessed August 1, 2008.

"could be a risk factor":

69   Daniel M. Sheehan, "Herbal Medicines, Phytoestrogens and Toxicity:
      Risk:Benefit Considerations," *Proceedings of the Society of Experimental
      Biology and Medicine,* 217, no. 3 (March 1998): 379–85, http://www.ncbi
      .nlm.nih.gov/pubmed/9492351.

excess production of estrogen:

69   Program on Breast Cancer and Environmental Risk Factors, Cornell Uni-
      versity, College of Veterinary Medicine, http://envirocancer.cornell.edu.

In boys, extra estrogen:

69   Laurence H. Klotz, "Why Is the Rate of Testicular Cancer Increasing?"
      Canadian Medical Association Journal (January 26, 1999): 160,
      http://www.cmaj.ca/cgi/reprint/160/2/213.pdf.

higher risk of breast or ovarian:

69   Program on Breast Cancer and Environmental Risk Factors, Cornell Uni-
      versity, College of Veterinary Medicine, http://envirocancer.cornell.edu.

"goitrogenic and even carcinogenic":

69   Sheehan, "Herbal Medicines, Phytoestrogens and Toxicity."

"all estrogens which have been studied":

70   Sheehan and Doerge, http://www.soyonlineservice.co.nz/downloads/
      nctrpti.pdf.

"The animal data":

70   Ibid.

In May–June 2000, an article:

70   John Henkel, "Soy: Health Claims for Soy Proteins, Questions About
      Other Components," *FDA Consumer* (May–June 2000), http://www.fda
      .gov/Fdac/features/2000/300_soy.html.

their concern that soy:

71   Daniel M. Sheehan and Daniel R. Doerge, "Goitrogenic and Estrogenic
      Activity of Soy Isoflavones," *Environmental Health Perspectives* 110,
      suppl. 3 (June 2002): 349–53.

"minimal or no benefit":

71   Frank M. Sacks et al., "Soy Protein, Isoflavones, and Cardiovascular
      Health," *Circulation* 113 (2006): 1034–44.

quietly withdrew:

71   Ibid.

"Against the backdrop":

71   Marian Burros, "Doubts Cloud Rosy News on Soy," *New York Times,* Jan-
      uary 26, 2000.

"You have to be soy careful":

72   *Washington Post* Health Section, January 30, 2001.

though CNN did mention:

72   Health: This Week in the Medical Journals, http://www.cnn.com/2006/
      HEALTH/01/26/journal.roundup/index.html.

tendency to block our absorption:

72   Bo Lönnerdal, Ann-Sofi Sandberg, Brittmarie Sandstrom, and Clemens
      Kunz, "Inhibitory Effects of Phytic Acid and Other Inositol Phosphates
      on Zinc and Calcium Absorption in Suckling Rats," *Mineral Trace and
      Elements,* American Institute of Nutrition, http://jn.nutrition.org/cgi/
      reprint/119/2/211.pdf, accessed August 1, 2008.

"These toxins that act":

73   Sally Fallon and Mary G. Enig, "Tragedy & Hype: The Third Interna-
      tional Soy Symposium," *Nexus* 7, no. 3 (April–May 2000). First published
      for "Wise Traditions" at the Weston A. Price Foundation, a nonprofit, tax-
      exempt charity founded in 1999 to disseminate the research of nutrition
      pioneer Dr. Weston Price, http://www.westonaprice.org/soy/tragedy.html.

"the mineral-blocking effects":

73   B. Sandstrom et al., "Effect of Protein Level and Protein Source on
      Zinc Absorption in Humans," *Journal of Nutrition* 119, no. 1 (January
      1989): 48–53; Susan Tait et al., "The Availability of Minerals in Food, with
      Particular Reference to Iron," *Journal of Research in Society and Health*
      103, no. 2 (April 1983): 74–77; cited by Fallon and Enig, "Tragedy &
      Hype."

pigs also have trouble:

73   Kimball Nill, "Correcting the Myths: Presenting the Truth About Why
      U.S. Farmers Have Adopted Biotechnology," the American Soybean
      Association, May 2003, http://www.data.forestry.oregonstate.edu/orb/
      Myths/Correcting_Myths.soy.pdf, accessed August 1, 2008.

"Instead of being digested":

74   Ibid.

"those animals consume":

74   Ibid.

"soy plays at least a small part":

75   GMO Compass, "Ingredients and Additives: Soy Is Everywhere," http://
      www.gmo-compass.org/eng/grocery_shopping/ingredients_additives/
      34.ingredients_additives_soybeans.html, accessed August 1, 2008.

soy lecithin:

75   U.S. Food and Drug Administration, Center for Food Safety and Applied
      Nutrition, Office of Food Additive Safety, April 2006, Guidance for In-
      dustry, Guidance on the Labeling of Certain Uses of Lecithin Derived
      from Soy Under Section 403(w) of the Federal Food, Drug, and Cos-
      metic Act, http://www.cfsan.fda.gov/~dms/soyguid.html.

there is some evidence:

75   Dan Ferber, "More Good News for Peanut Allergy Sufferers," *Science-
      NOW,* March 10, 2003, p. 2; Kathryn Scott, "Soy Sensitive, A Guide to
      Soy Allergy and Intolerance," *Living Without* (Summer 2007),
      http://www.livingwithout.com/2007/sum07soy.html:

To complicate matters further, soy goes by many other names: diglyc-
eride, edamame, glycine max, hydrolyzed vegetable protein (HVP),
lecithin, miso, monoglyceride, monosodium glutamate (MSG), natto,
tamari, tempeh, tofu, vegetable oil, vitamin E, and yuba.

FALCPA has helped clarify the confusion somewhat. Since January 1, 2006, food manufacturers are required to clearly state on food
labels if soy, or any one of the other eight most common allergens, is
one of the ingredients.

However, even with the new law in place, it's still important to read
labels carefully. The law doesn't apply to non-food items like cosmetics and medicine. And according to the FDA, FALCPA doesn't require food manufacturers or retailers to re-label or remove products
with the old labeling as long as they were labeled before January 1,
2006. As a result the FDA warns shoppers of ". . . a transition period
of undetermined length during which it is likely that consumers will
see packaged food on store shelves and in consumers' homes without
the revised allergen labeling."

Hydrolized soy protein:

76   GMO Compass, "Ingredients and Additives: Soy Is Everywhere"; U.S. Food and Drug Administration, Guidance on the Labeling of Certain Uses of Lecithin Derived from Soy.

Soy can also be found in MSG:

76   K. He et al., "Association of Monosodium Glutamate Intake with Overweight in Chinese Adults: The INTERMAP Study," *Obesity* 16, no. 8, (2008): 1875–80; Ferber, "More Good News for Peanut Allergy Sufferers."

A 1997 study:

76   K. D. Setchell et al., "Exposure of Infants to Phyto-oestrogens from Soy-based Infant Formula," *Lancet* 350, no. 9080 (September 13, 1997): 815–16, http://www.ncbi.nlm.nih.gov/pubmed/9217716.

Among girls and women:

77   Janet Gray, "State of the Evidence 2008: The Connection Between Breast Cancer and the Environment," http://www.breastcancerfund.org/site/apps/nlnet/content.aspx?c=kwKXLdPaE&b=86186&content_id={41D4559D-4539-469A-B36F-8ECB33C967F1}&notoc=1.

And when males are overexposed:

77   Ibid.

"a large, uncontrolled":

77   Mike Fitzpatrick, "Dangers of Dietary Isoflavones at Levels Above Those Found in Traditional Diets," http://www.westonaprice.org/soy/isoflavones.html.

the British medical establishment:

77   Institute of Food Research, UK, Soya Information Sheet, http://www.ifr.ac.uk/public/FoodInfoSheets/soya.html.

"[s]oy protein is a potential allergen":

77   Pat Tuohy, "Soy-Based Formula" (December 1998), http://www.moh.govt.nz/moh.nsf/Files/mohsoy/$file/mohsoy.pdf.

In 2005, the Israeli:

77 *Soy and Health* 8 (September 2005), http://www.soyconference.com/magazines/sep05.pdf, August 1, 2008.

In 2006, the French Food Agency:

78 Sébastien Vergne et al., "Bioavailability and Urinary Excretion of Isoflavones in Humans: Effects of Soy-based Supplements Formulation and Equol Production," *Journal of Pharmaceutical and Biomedical Analysis* 43, no. 4 (March 12, 2007); J. Mathey et al., "Concentrations of Isoflavones in Plasma and Urine of Post-menopausal Women Chronically Ingesting High Quantities of Soy Isoflavones." *Journal of Pharmaceutical and Biomedical Analysis* 41, no. 3 (June 7, 2006): 41.

In November 2007, the Germans:

78 Federal Institute for Risk Assessment, "Isolated Isoflavones Are Not Without Risk," http://www.bfr.bund.de/cm/245/isolated_isoflavones_are_not_without_risk.pdf, accessed August 1, 2008.

Dr. William Sears:

78 Bottle Feeding Index, http://www.askdrsears.com/html/0/T000100.asp, accessed August 1, 2008.

"There is no precedent":

78 Ibid.

"Giving an infant soy":

79 Ibid.

"Soy protein–based":

79 Jatinder Bhatia and Frank Greer, "Use of Soy Protein–Based Formulas in Infant Feeding," *Pediatrics* 121, no. 5 (May 2008): 1062–68. See also Vincent Iannelli, "Pediatrics: Soy Milk and Soy Baby Formula, Child Nutrition Basics," http://pediatrics.about.com/od/infantformula/a/0508_soy_milk.htm.

an enormous chemical corporation:

80 Tom Philpott, "Dominant Traits: Monsanto's Latest Court Triumph Cloaks Massive Market Power," *Grist, Environmental News and Com-*

mentary, January 17, 2008, http://www.grist.org/comments/food/2008/ 01/17/, accessed August 1, 2008.

tragic results for several children:

80   T. Foucard, I. Malmheden, and I. Yman, "A Study on Severe Food Reactions in Sweden: Is Soy Protein an Underestimated Cause of Food Anaphylaxis?" *Allergy* 54, no. 3 (2001): 261–65.

scientific papers about the condition:

81   S. H. Sicherer, Hugh A. Sampson, and A. W. Burks, "Peanut and Soy Allergy: A Clinical and Therapeutic Dilemma," *Allergy* 55, no. 6 (2000): 515–21.

genetically engineered protein:

81   U.S. Patent 7381556, Nucleic acids encoding deallergenized proteins and permuteins. Inventors: Murtaza F. Alibhai, James D. Astwood, Charles A. McWherter, Hugh A. Sampson. Assignee: Monsanto Technology, LLC. Issued by the United States Patent and Trademark Office, June 3, 2008. Patent Storm, http://www.patentstorm.us/patents/ 7381556.html, accessed July 8, 2008.

relationship between allergies:

81   Sicherer, Sampson, and Burks, "Peanut and Soy Allergy."

FAAN went ballistic:

82   Food Allergy and Anaphylaxis Network, "Will Soy Cause a Reaction in Someone with Peanut Allergy?" http://www.foodallergy.org/media/ HotTopics/SoyPeanut.html, accessed August 1, 2008.

"If your child is allergic":

82   Foucard, Malmheden, and Yman, "A Study on Severe Food Reactions in Sweden."

"Some sensitive children":

82   Ibid., and AllergyKids, "Soy's Cross Reactivity in Children with Asthma and Allergy," April 20, 2007, http://www.allergykids.com/index.php ?id=4&page=Our_Research.

basically told parents:

83   Food Allergy and Anaphylaxis Network, "Will Soy Cause a Reaction in
      Someone with Peanut Allergy?"

a 2005 Finnish study:

83   Timo Klemola et al., "Feeding a Soy Formula to Children with Cow's Milk
      Allergy: The Development of Immunoglobulin E–mediated Allergy to Soy
      and Peanuts," *Pediatric Allergy and Immunology* 16, no. 8 (2005): 641–46.

a 1999 U.S. study:

83   R. S. Zeiger, H. A. Sampson, and S. A. Bock et al., "Soy Allergy in Infants
      and Children with IgE-associated Cow's Milk Allergy." *Journal of Pedi-
      atrics* 134, no. 5 (1999): 614–22.

"although most infants":

84   Jatinder Bhatia, Frank Greer, and the Committee on Nutrition, "Use of
      Soy Protein–based Formulas in Infant Feeding," *Pediatrics* 121, no. 5
      (May 2008): 1062–68.

The British study:

84   Gideon Lack et al., "Factors Associated with the Development of Peanut
      Allergy in Childhood," *New England Journal of Medicine* 348, 11 (March
      13, 2003): 977–85.

allergies from the skin creams:

85   Ibid.

Dr. Paul Kuwayama:

85   "Peanut Allergies Linked to Soy Formula," NBC 4, Washington D.C.
      Metro Area, November 13, 2002, http://www.nbc4.com/health/1783187/
      detail.html, accessed August 1, 2008.

265 percent increase:

86   Amy M. Branum and Susan L. Lukacs, "Food Allergy Among U.S. Chil-
      dren: Trends in Prevalence and Hospitalizations," NCHS Data Brief no.
      10, October 2008, http://www.cdc.gov/nchs/data/databriefs/db10.pdf;
      Centers for Disease Control, "CDC Study Finds 3 Million U.S. Chil-
      dren Have Food or Digestive Allergies," October 22, 2008, http://
      www.cdc.gov/media/pressrel/2008/r081022.htm.

"additional study":

86   Bhatia and Greer, "Use of Soy Protein–based Formulas in Infant
      Feeding."

twelve genetically engineered (GE) plant species:

87   Genetically Engineered Organisms—Public Issues Education Project,
      "What Traits Have Been Engineered?" Cornell University, http://www
      .geo-pie.cornell.edu/traits/traits.html, accessed August 1, 2008.

quotes James D. Astwood:

88   Beatrice Trum Hunter, "Food Allergies: No Trivial Health Matter," *Con-
      sumers' Research Magazine* (February 1, 1999).

proteins from the Brazil nut:

89   Genetically Engineered Organisms—Public Issues Education Project,
      Cornell University, "Case Study: Brazil Nut Allergen in GE Soybeans,"
      http://www.geo-pie.cornell.edu/issues/brazilnut.html, accessed August 1,
      2008.

According to the article:

90   Smith, *Seeds of Deception,* p. 160.

The committee's task:

90   Notes from the Food Biotechnology Subcommittee meeting of the Food
      Advisory Committee, held August 13, 2002, by the Department of Health
      and Human Services, Food and Drug Administration, and Center
      for Food Safety and Applied Nutrition, http://www.fda.gov/OHRMS/
      DOCKETS/ac/02/transcripts/3886t1.doc, accessed August 1, 2008.

In response to a discussion:

90   Ibid.

"the logical problem":

91   Ibid.

A July 27, 2004, report:

92   Netherwood et al., "Assessing the Survival of Transgenic Plant DNA in
      the Human Gastrointestinal Tract," *Nature Biotechnology* 22 (2004).

Dr. Irina Ermakova:

92   Geoffrey Lean, "Mortality Rate for New-born Rats Six Times Higher When Mother Was Fed on a Diet of Modified Soya," *The Independent,* January 8, 2006, http://www.independent.co.uk/environment/gm-new -study-shows-unborn-babies-could-be-harmed-522109.html.

"secret report":

92   Geoffrey Lean, "Revealed: Health Fears Over Secret Study into GM Food, Rats Fed GM Corn Due for Sale in Britain Developed Abnormalities in Blood and Kidneys," *The Independent,* May 22, 2005, http://www.independent.co.uk/news/science/revealed-health-fears-over -secret-study-into-gm-food-491657.html.

Chapter 4. Milk Money

Health and Human Services workshop:

96   Assessment of the Allergenic Potential of Genetically Modified Foods, December 10–12, 2001, Chapel Hill, N.C. Sponsored by the Office of Research and Development, U.S. Environmental Protection Agency, National Toxicology Program, Department of Health and Human Services, National Institute of Environmental Health Sciences, National Institutes of Health Office of Rare Diseases, National Institutes of Health Center for Food Safety and Nutrition, U.S. Food and Drug Administration. Organized by the National Institute of Environmental Health Sciences National Toxicology Program. http://ntp-server.niehs.nih.gov/ntp/htdocs/ Liaison/Allergenicity.pdf, accessed August 1, 2008.

the review article:

96   S. H. Sicherer, Hugh A. Sampson, and A. W. Burks, "Peanut and Soy Allergy: A Clinical and Therapeutic Dilemma," *Allergy* 55, no. 6 (2000): 515–21.

GM-related scandal:

96   United States Environmental Protection Agency, Scientific Advisory Panel Meeting, July 13, 2001, http://www.epa.gov/scipoly/sap/meetings/ 2001/july/agenda.htm, accessed August 1, 2008.

This giant agrichemical:

97   Vote Yes on Measure 27, The Monsanto Files, http://www.voteyeson27
       .com/monsanto.htm, accessed August 1, 2008.

the company is worth:

97   CNNMoney.com, http://money.cnn.com/quote/quotehtml?symb=MON,
       accessed June 2008.

Now the Associated Press:

98   Christopher Leonard, "Monsanto Sells Controversial Cow Hormone
       for $300 Million, Posilac Cow Hormone Receives Attention Because
       of Health Concerns," August 21, 2008, http://www.statesman.com/
       business/content/business/stories/other/08/21/0821monsanto.html;
       "Monsanto Sells Controversial Posilac Cow Hormone to Eli Lilly for $300
       Million," *Business Week,* August 20, 2008, http://investing.businessweek
       .com/research/stocks/news/article.asp?docKey=600-200808202305INV
       TRENDFINANCE_89507-3QDR6O0JFB7ODPK97FS4HKIVC1
       &params=timestamp%7C%7C08/20/2008%2011:05%20PM%20ET%7C
       %7Cheadline%7C%7CMonsanto%20Sells%20Controversial%20Posilac
       %20Cow%20Hormone%20To%20Eli%20Lilly%20For%20%24300%20
       Million%7C%7CdocSource%7C%7CInvestrend%7C%7Cprovider%7C
       %7CACQUIREMEDIA& symbol=JNJ; Andrew Martin and Andrew Pol-
       lack, "Monsanto Looks to Sell Dairy Hormone Business," *New York
       Times,* August 8, 2008, http://www.nytimes.com/2008/08/07business/
       07bovine.html?_r=1&ref=health&oref=slogin; "Eli Lilly to Buy Mon-
       santo's Dairy Cow Hormone for $300 Million," *New York Times,* August
       20, 2008, http://dealbook.blogs.nytimes.com/2008/08/20/eli-lilly-to-buy
       -monsantos-dairy-cow-hormone-for-300-million/?scp=2&sq=monsanto
       %20posilac&st=cse.

So what is rBGH:

98   Suemedha Sood, "Milking It, Why Monsanto Doesn't Want You to Know
       About Those Hormones in Your Dairy," *Washington Independent,* March
       25, 2008, http://www.washingtonindependent.com/view/milking-it.

about one-third of the nation's cows:

98   Laura Sayre, "Protecting Milk from Monsanto, Don't Let Corporate
       Interests Trump Your Right to Know What's in the Milk You Drink,"
       Mother Earth News, June/July 2008, http://www.motherearthnews

.com/Sustainable-Farming/2008-06-01/Artificial-Hormones-Milk.aspx;
Sood, "Milking It."

"essentially all . . . *milk"*:
99   Becky Gillette, "Doin' a Body Good? Studies Link rBGH-Produced Milk
        and Increased Cancer Risk," *E Magazine,* http://www.emagazine.com/
        view/?1006last, accessed June 7, 2008.

milk allergy:
100   Sharona Schwartz, "Study: Milk Allergy Can Take Years Longer to Out-
        grow," http://www.cnn.com/2007/HEALTH/conditions/11/12/milk.allergy/
        index.html, accessed June 7, 2008.

"risk of clinical lameness":
100   Food Animal Concerns Trust, "What Is Happening to Dairy Cows? An
        Emerging Area of Farm Animal Abuse and Public Health Risk,"
        http://web.archive.org/web/20061002004733/; http://www.foodanimal
        concernstrust.org/dairycows.htm.

cows hopped-up on rBGH:
100   Health Canada, Report of the Canadian Veterinary Medical Association
        Expert Panel on rBST, p. 11, http://www.hc-sc.gc.ca/dhp-mps/vct/
        issues-enjeux/rbst-stbr/rcp_cvma-rap_acdv_09-eng.php.

Codex Alimentarius:
100   Donald L. Barlett and James B. Steele, "Investigation: Monsanto's
        Harvest of Fear," *Vanity Fair,* May 2008, http://www.vanityfair.com/
        politics/features/2008/05/monsanto200805.

25 to 40 percent of dairy farmers:
101   Sayre, "Protecting Milk from Monsanto."

Other farmers have said:
101   Sood, "Milking It."

dairy program subsidies:
101   Environmental Working Group, Dairy Program Subsidies in the
        United States, http://farm.ewg.org/farm/progdetail.php?fips=00000
        &progcode=dairy, accessed June 7, 2008.

"More milk means":

101 Sood, "Milking It."

As early as 1998:

102 R. W. Furlaneto and I. N. DiCarlo, "New Study Warns of Breast and Colon Cancer Risk of rBGH Milk," *Cancer Research* 44 (1984): 2122–28; P. Gregor and B. D. Burleigh, "Presence of High Affinity Somatomedin/Insulin-line Growth Factor Receptors in Porcine Mammary Gland," *Endocrinology* 116, suppl. 1 (1985): 223; P. G. Campbell and C. R. Baumrucker, "Characterization of Insulin-like Growth Factor-1/Somatomedin-C Receptors in Bovine Mammary Gland," *Endocrinology* 116, suppl. 1 (1985): 223, http://www.preventcancer.com/press/conference/jan23_96.htm.

According to a January 1996:

102 Hans R. Larsen, "Milk and the Cancer Connection," *International Health News* 76 (April 1998), http://www.notmilk.com/drlarsen.html.

More recent studies:

102 Samuel S. Epstein, Petition Letter to United States Department of Health and Human Services Seeking the Withdrawal of the New Animal Drug Application Approval for Posilac—Recombinant Bovine Growth Hormone (rBGH), February 15, 2007, http://www.prevent cancer.com/publications/pdf/Petition_Posilac_feb 157.pdf.

one in 229 women:

102 Statistics from the Young Survival Coalition, http://www.youngsurvival .org/young-women-and-bc/statistic.

one in eight women:

102 Breast Cancer Fund, Eliminating the Environmental Causes of Breast Cancer, http://www.breastcancerfund.org/site/pp.asp?c=kwKXLdPaE&b =43969.

prostate and colon cancer:

102 Sood, "Milking It."

"It's been known for years":

103 Ibid.

regulates the release:

103   Judith Collier et al., *Oxford Handbook of Clinical Specialties,* 7th ed. (Oxford, 2006), pp. 350–51.

As Dr. Pompilio explains:

103   Sood, "Milking It."

"In this area":

103   Kurt Eichenwald, Gina Kolata, and Melody Petersen, "Redesigning Nature: Hard Lessons Learned; Biotechnology Food: From the Lab to a Debacle," *New York Times,* January 25, 2001, http://query.nytimes .com/gst/fullpage.html?res=9903E1D8163FF936A15752C0A9679C8 B63&sec=health&spon=&pagewanted=5).

"Ultimately, it is the food producer":

103   Food and Drug Administration, "Statement of Policy: Foods Derived from New Plant Varieties" (GMO Policy), *Federal Register* 57, no. 104 (1992): 229.

"Monsanto should not have to":

104   Michael Pollan, "Playing God in the Garden," *New York Times Magazine,* October 25, 1998, http://query.nytimes.com/gst/fullpage.html?res =9D03EFD8143DF936A15753C1A96E958260&sec=&spon=&page wanted=12.

Why did the FDA:

105   Source Watch, "Labeling Issues, Revolving Doors, rBGH, Bribery and Monsanto," http://www.sourcewatch.org/index.php?title=Labeling _Issues%2C_Revolving_Doors%2C_rBGH%2C_Bribery_and_Monsanto, accessed August 4, 2008.

Monsanto's law firm:

105   Jennifer Ferrara, "Revolving Doors: Monsanto and the Regulators," http://www.monitor.net/monitor/9904b/monsantofda.html, excerpted from "The Monsanto Files, Can We Survive Genetic Engineering?" *The Ecologist* 28, no. 5 (September 1998); Source Watch, "Labeling Issues, Revolving Doors."

a new position for Taylor:

105   Jeffrey M. Smith, *Seeds of Deception, Exposing Government Lies About the Safety of the Genetically Engineered Foods You're Eating* (Yes! Books, 2003), p. 83.

Miller probably felt:

106   Ibid.

According to the GAO:

106   Ferrara, "Revolving Doors"; Source Watch, "Labeling Issues, Revolving Doors."

they went after Oakhurst:

107   Matt Wickenheiser, "Oakhurst Sued by Monsanto Over Milk Advertising," *Portland Press Herald,* July 8, 2003, http://www.pressherald.com/news/local/030708oakhurst.shtml.

Meanwhile, Monsanto:

107   "Federal Agencies Advised of Misleading Milk Labels and Advertising," *PR Newswire,* April 3, 2007, http://www.prnewswire.com/cgi-bin/stories .pl?ACCT=104&STORY=/www/story/04-03-2007/0004558844 &EDATE, accessed August 4, 2008.

"no consumer research":

108   Andrew Martin, "Fighting on a Battlefield the Size of a Milk Label," *New York Times,* March 9, 2008, http://www.nytimes.com/2008/03/09/business/09feed.html?adxnnl=1&adxnnlx=1212901207-Vh1Dj0xR fjKMrGm51NytJw.

Consumer Reports:

108   Center for Food Safety Press Release, "90 Consumer, Environmental Groups and Dairies Urge Utah to Not Ban Milk Hormone Labeling; Recent Similar Attempts to Ban rBGH-Free Labels in Other States Have Failed," February 25, 2008; Michael Hansen, "Pennsylvania Reverses Decision on Milk Labeling," *Consumer Reports,* January 23, 2008, http://blogs.consumerreports.org/safety/2008/01milk-hormone -la.html.

Osborn & Barr:

108   Martin, "Fighting on a Battlefield the Size of a Milk Label."

Monsanto also contributes:

108   Ibid.

Center for Consumer Freedom:

108   Source Watch, a Project for the Center of Media and Democracy, Center for Consumer Freedom, http://www.sourcewatch.org/index.php?title =Center_for_Consumer_Freedom, accessed August 4, 2008.

"Dr. Evil":

109   Deirdre Naphin and Katy Textor, "Meet Rick Berman, AKA 'Dr. Evil,' Morley Safer Speaks to a Lobbyist Some People Love to Hate," CBS News/*60 Minutes,* July 22, 2007, http://www.cbsnews.com/stories/2007/ 04/05/60minutes/main2653020.shtml.

"Most of the nation's":

109   Sood, "Milking It."

Of the 100 top:

109   Sayre, "Protecting Milk from Monsanto."

Roundup wasn't the first:

110   Barlett and Steele, "Investigation: Monsanto's Harvest of Fear."

Robert Shapiro:

111   Ibid.

GM products spread:

111   United States Department of Agriculture, Economic Research Service, "The Economics of Food, Farming, Natural Resources and Rural America, Adoption of Genetically Engineered Crops in the U.S.: Corn Varieties," updated July 2, 2008, http://www.ers.usda.gov/Data/BiotechCrops/ ExtentofAdoptionTable1.htm; "Adoption of Genetically Engineered Crops in the U.S.: Soybeans Varieties," http://www.ers.usda.gov/Data/ BiotechCrops/ExtentofAdoptionTable3.htm, accessed August 4, 2008; Brendan I. Koerner, "How Much of Our Food Is Bioengineered?" *Slate,* May 22, 2003, http://www.slate.com/id/2083482/.

Monsanto comes after you:

112 Paul Elias, "Enforcing Single Season Seeds, Monsanto Sues Farmers," January 13, 2005, http://www.usatoday.com/tech/news/2005-01-13 -biotech-pirates_x.htm.

"As interviews and reams":

112 Barlett and Steele, "Investigation: Monsanto's Harvest of Fear."

Monsanto made the most:

113 Ibid.

Chapter 5. Corn Controversies

Michael Pollan's book:

119 Michael Pollan, *The Omnivore's Dilemma* (Penguin Books, 2006).

corn lurks in places:

119 Judy Ciarcia Keller, "Corn Allergic or Crazy, Seeking a Kernel of Truth," *Living Without,* http://www.livingwithout.com/features/vault_corncrazy .html.

corn allergy does exist:

120 Ibid.

FDA should catch up:

120 Ibid.

simply underdiagnosed:

120 Ibid.

"Bt has been available":

121 Ric Bessin, "Bt Corn, What It Is and How It Works," University of Kentucky College of Agriculture, http://www.ca.uky.edu/entomology/ entfacts/efl30.asp.

121 The material on pages 121–142 is based on an interview with Michael K. Hansen, PhD, senior staff scientist, Consumers Union, conducted on May 29, 2008, except where specific documents are cited.

new insect-resistant Bt cotton:

129   Ibid.

In 2003, eleven:

129   Ibid.

In 2005, a researcher:

129   Ibid.

The StarLink scandal:

131   "StarLink: GE Corn in Taco Shells, Genetically Engineered Organisms,"
Public Issues Education Project, Cornell University, http://www.geo-ie
.cornell.edu/issues/starlink.html.

into the beer supply:

131   Joseph Levitt, director, Center for Food Safety, quoted on Monsanto's
Web site, http://www.monsanto.co.uk/achievements/00/canola.html:
"Biotechnology in and of itself does not make a product different." "FDA
also has identified the presence of StarLink corn, by both protein and
DNA testing, in a corn meal product marketed to the brewing industry,'
Joseph Levitt, director of the FDA's center for food safety, revealed in a let-
ter to Senator Durbin after the FDA had analyzed 129 U.S. food samples.
The letter was also signed by Jim Aidala, an EPA assistant administrator,
and by Enrique Figueroa, a USDA deputy undersecretary," *Los Angeles
Times,* January 18, 2001, http://www.mindfully.org/GE/StarLinked-Beer
.htm, accessed August 1, 2008.

The government agencies:

132   Andrew Pollack, "U.S. Finds No Allergies to Altered Corn," *New York
Times,* June 14, 2001, http://query.nytimes.com/gst/fullpage.html
?res=9A0CE4DC1F3EF937A25755C0A9679C8B63.

The EPA panel:

132   "StarLink: GE Corn in Taco Shells."

"Although StarLink corn":

132   Ibid.

"[N]obody can say":

133   Nutrition Action Healthletter, "Genetically Engineered Allergies?" (April 2001), Center for Science in the Public Interest, http://www.cspinet .org/nah/04_01/index.html.

Dr. Sampson had gone on to develop:

133   U.S. Patent 7381556, Nucleic acids encoding deallergenized proteins and permuteins. Inventors: Murtaza F. Alibhai, James D. Astwood, Charles A. McWherter, Hugh A. Sampson. Assignee: Monsanto Technology, LLC. Issued by the United States Patent and Trademark Office, June 3, 2008. Patent Storm, http://www.patentstorm.us/patents/7381556.html, accessed July 8, 2008.

The seventeen people tested:

133   "StarLink: GE Corn in Taco Shells"; Bill Freese, "The StarLink Affair: A Critique of the Government/Industry Response to Contamination of the Food Supply with StarLink Corn and an Examination of the Potential Allergenicity of StarLink's Cry9C Protein, for Submission to the FIFRA Scientific Advisory Panel Considering Assessment of Additional Scientific Information Concerning StarLink™ Corn," July 17–19, 2001. Docket Control No. OPP-00724; also for submission to Docket Control No. PF-1029.

critics claimed that the test results:

134   "Scientific Critique of FDA Whitewash of Starlink Corn Allergy Scandal," Genetically Engineered Food Alert, Scientific Advisory Panel transcript, p. 461, http://www.organicconsumers.org/gefood/fdaallergyscandal.cfm; Freese, "The StarLink Affair"; Pollack, "U.S. Finds No Allergies to Altered Corn."

Health hazards don't affect:

134   "Scientific Critique of FDA Whitewash of Starlink Corn Allergy Scandal"; Freese, "The StarLink Affair."

Children's health was a special concern:

135   Jatinder Bhatia, Frank Greer, and the Committee on Nutrition, "Use of Soy Protein–based Formulas in Infant Feeding," *Pediatrics* 121, no. 5 (May 2008): 1062–68.

Mead Johnson's Enfamil Nutramigen:
135   Freese, "The StarLink Affair."

Another vulnerable group:
135   Ibid.

"Reasons for Caution":
136   Hansen interview.

part of that deregulation process:
136   Kurt Eichenwald, Gina Kolata, and Melody Petersen, "Redesigning Na-
       ture: Hard Lessons Learned; Biotechnology Food: From the Lab to a
       Debacle," *New York Times,* January 25, 2001, http://query.nytimes.com/
       gst/fullpage.html?res=9903E1D8163FF936A15752C0A9679C8B63
       &sec=health&spon=&pagewanted=5.

"This is the industry's pet":
137   Ibid.

"The possibility of unexpected":
137   Ibid.

A series of studies:
139   Michael Hansen, "Reasons for Caution About Introducing Genetically
       Engineered Corn in Africa: Food Safety Issues," unpublished paper, pro-
       vided courtesy of the author.

Joe Cummins, professor emeritus:
139   Hansen interview.

bee populations declined:
141   Lora A. Morandin and Mark L. Winston, "Wild Bee Abundance and Seed
       Production in Conventional, Organic, and Genetically Modified Canola,"
       Ecological Applications 15, no. 3 (2005): 871–81.

cows fed on genetically modified fodder:
142   Hansen interview.

firestorm of bad publicity:

142   Andy Rees, "GM Potatoes—Facts and Fictions," *The Ecologist,* Sep-
       tember 22, 2006, http://www.theecologist.org/pages/archive_detail.asp
       ?content_id=612.

Chapter 6. True Colors

Dr. Bock describes:

150   Kenneth Bock, *Healing the New Childhood Epidemics: Autism, ADHD,
       Asthma and Allergies* (Random House, 2007).

the Feingold Association:

152   Feingold Association of the United States, http://www.feingold.org.

Researchers at Southampton University:

153   D. McCann et al., "Food Additives and Hyperactive Behaviour in 3-year-
       old and 8/9-year-old Children in the Community: A Randomised,
       Double-blinded, Placebo-controlled Trial," *The Lancet* 370, no. 9598
       (November 3, 2007): 1524–25.

"[P]arents should not think":

154   Ibid.

As early as April 24, 1988:

154   K. S. Rowe, "Synthetic Food Colourings and 'Hyperactivity': A Double-
       blind Crossover Study," *Australian Paediatric Journal* 24, no. 2 (April
       1988): 143–47.

"a significant effect":

156   C. M. Carter et al., "Effects of a Few Foods Diet in Attention Deficit
       Disorder," *Archives of Disease in Childhood* 69, no. 5 (November 1993):
       564–68.

the study concerned some 200 children:

157   K. S. Rowe and K. J. Rowe, "Synthetic Food Coloring and Behavior: A
       Dose Response Effect in a Double-blind, Placebo-controlled, Repeated-
       Measures Study," *Australian Paediatric Journal* 135 (November 1994):
       691–98.

elevated levels of eosinophils:

158   I. L. D. Moutinho, L. C. Bertges, and R. V. C. Assis, "Prolonged Use of
      the Food Dye Tartrazine (FD&C Yellow no. 5) and Its Effects on the Gas-
      tric Mucosa of Wistar Rats," *Brazilian Journal of Biology* 67 (February
      2007); "Eosinophilic Disorders Homepage," Cincinnati Children's Hos-
      pital Medical Center, www.cincinnatichildrens.org/svc/prog/eosinophilic/
      patients.htm, accessed November 26, 2004.

"allergic reactions to food colors":

158   J. A. Mattes and R. Gittelman, "Effects of Artificial Food Colorings in
      Children with Hyperactive Symptoms. A Critical Review and Results of
      a Controlled Study," *Archives of General Psychiatry* 38, no. 6 (June 1981):
      714–18.

"From 4% to 14%":

158   M. E. MacCara, "Tartrazine: A Potentially Hazardous Dye in Canadian
      Drugs," *Canadian Medical Association Journal* 126, no. 8 (April 15, 1982):
      910–14.

a previous study in 2004:

158   B. Bateman et al., "The Effects of a Double-blind, Placebo-controlled, Ar-
      tificial Food Colourings and Benzoate Preservative Challenge on Hyper-
      activity in a General Population Sample of Preschool Children," *Archives
      of Disease in Childhood* 89, no. 6 (June 2004): 506–11.

an Australian study:

159   Andrew Kemp, "Food Additives and Hyperactivity: Evidence Supports a
      Trial Period of Eliminating Colourings and Preservatives from the Diet,"
      British Medical Journal 336, no. 1144 (May 24, 2008).

most children need far more sleep:

160   Seung-Schik Yoo et al., "The Human Emotional Brain Without Sleep: A
      Prefrontal-Amygdala Disconnect," *Current Biology* 17 (2007): 877–78; Po
      Bronson, "Snooze or Lose," *New York Magazine,* October 15, 2007, p. 34.

lots of factors involved:

160   D. A. Christakis et al., "Early Television Exposure and Subsequent At-
      tentional Problems in Children," *Pediatrics* 113 (2004): 708–13.

Thomas Spencer, MD:

161   Elisabeth Rosenthal, "Some Food Additives Raise Hyperactivity, Study Finds," *New York Times,* September 6, 2007, http://www.nytimes.com/2007/09/06/health/research/06hyper.html?_r=1&adxnnl=1&oref=slogin&adxnnlx=1217956872-TTaFbbT5A1/IwBExn6K5Ew.

Aspartame has been linked:

162   J. W. Olney et al., "Increasing Brain Tumor Rates: Is There a Link to Aspartame?" *Journal of Neuropathology and Experimental Neurology* 55, no. 11 (November 1996): 1115–23.

Fourteen years later:

162   Andrew Cockburn, *Rumsfeld: His Rise, Fall, and Catastrophic Legacy* (Simon and Schuster, 2007), pp. 63–64.

human and animal studies:

162   T. J. Maher and R. J. Wurtman, "Possible Neurologic Effects of Aspartame, a Widely Used Food Additive," *Environmental Health Perspectives* 75 (November 1987): 53–57; G. Guiso et al., "Effect of Aspartame on Seizures in Various Models of Experimental Epilepsy," *Toxicology and Applied Pharmacology* 96, no. 3 (December 1988): 485–93; C. Trocho et al., "Formaldehyde Derived from Dietary Aspartame Binds to Tissue Components in Vivo," *Life Sciences* 63, no. 5 (1998): 337–49, cited on the National Center for Biotechnology Information Web site, http://www.ncbi.nlm.nih.gov/pubmed/9714421.

David Ludwig, MD:

162   David Ludwig, personal communication, May 6, 2008.

"41 percent increase":

163   Sharon P. Fowler and Leslie Bonci, WebMD News: T. L. Davidson, "Artificial Sweeteners May Damage Diet Efforts," *International Journal of Obesity* 28 (July 2004): 933–55; CBS News, "Diet Soda Drinkers Gain Weight; Overweight Risk Soars 41 Percent with Each Daily Can of Diet Soda," June 13, 2005, http://www.cbsnews.com/stories/2005/06/13/health/webmd/main701408.shtml, accessed August 5, 2008.

"paradoxic weight gain":

163   W. C. Monte, "Aspartame: Methanol and Public Health," *Journal of Applied Nutrition* 36 (1984): 52.

women who were dieting:

163   J. H. Lavin, S. J. French, and N. W. Read, "The Effect of Sucrose- and Aspartame-sweetened Drinks on Energy Intake, Hunger and Food Choice of Female, Moderately Restrained Eaters," *International Journal of Obesity* 21, no. 1 (January 1997): 37–42.

long-term memory lapses:

163   Peter Rebhahn, "Dangerous Diet Drinks: Can't Live Without Your Diet Soda? It Might Be Worse for You Than You Think. Aspartame Can Wreak Havoc on Your Long-Term Memory" *Psychology Today Magazine* (March–April 2001).

people who develop brain tumors:

163   H. J. Roberts, "Does Aspartame Cause Human Brain Cancer," *Journal of Advancement in Medicine* 4, no. 4 (1991): 231–41; CBS News/*60 Minutes,* "How Sweet Is It?: Controversy Continues Over the Safety of Aspartame as FDA Widens Its Approval to Other Foods," December 29, 1996; J. W. Olney et al., "Increasing Brain Tumor Rates: Is There a Link to Aspartame?" *Journal of Neuropathology and Experimental Neurology* 55, no. 11 (November 1996).

long-term Italian study:

163   Morando Soffritti et al., "First Experimental Demonstration of the Multipotential Carcinogenic Effects of Aspartame Administered in the Feed to Sprague-Dawley Rats," *Environmental Health Perspectives* 114, no. 3 (2006): 379–85.

A 2005 follow-up:

163   Ibid.

subject of controversy:

164   European Food Safety Authority, Opinion of the Scientific Panel on food additives, flavourings, processing aids and materials in contact with food (AFC) related to a new long-term carcinogenicity study on aspartame. Question number: EFSA-Q-2005-122. Adopted date: March 5, 2006,

http://www.efsa.europa.eu/EFSA/efsa_locale-1178620753812
_1178620765743.htm; United States Food and Drug Administration,
FDA Statement on European Aspartame Study, May 8, 2006,
http://www.fda.gov/bbs/topics/NEWS/2006/NEW01369.html.

"significant shortcomings":

164 New Zealand Food Safety Authority, Food Safety Authority challenges
activists' views on aspartame, August 3, 2007, http://www.nzfsa.govt
.nz/publications/media-releases/2007/aspartame-activists-3-8-2007.htm,
accessed August 5, 2008.

criticizing the study:

164 Ibid.

the NCI concluded:

164 Marilynn Marchione, "No Cancer Risk Found in Diet Soda's Aspartame,"
Seattle Post Intelligencer, April 5, 2006, http://seattlepi.nwsource.com/
national/265559_soda05.html, accessed August 5, 2008.

"The greatest risk":

164 "Dr. Blaylock: Aspartame Is Still Hazardous," Newsmax.com, April 12,
2006, http://archive.newsmax.com/archives/articles/2006/4/12/104518
.shtml.

100 percent of those funded:

164 CBS News/60 *Minutes,* "How Sweet Is It?"

its own revolving door:

165 Ralph G. Walton, "Survey of Aspartame Studies: Correlation of Outcome
and Funding Sources," http://www.neoucom.edu/DEPTS/Psychiatry/
walton.htm.

"Funding source was significantly related":

165 L. I. Lesser et al., "Relationship Between Funding Source and Conclusion among Nutrition-related Scientific Articles," *Public Library of
Science Medicine* 4, no. 1 (2007): 5, as cited on the National Center
for Biotechnology Information Web site, http://www.ncbi.nlm.nih.gov/
pubmed/17214504?ordinalpos=2&itool=EntrezSystem2.PEntrez.Pubmed
.Pubmed_ResultsPanel.Pubmed_RVDocSum.

A 1998 Spanish study:

166   Trocho, "Formaldehyde Derived from Dietary Aspartame Binds to Tissue Components in Vivo."

Industry scientists:

166   H. H. Butchko et al., Medical and Scientific Affairs, The NutraSweet Company, "Aspartame: Review of Safety," *Regulatory Toxicology and Pharmacology* 35, no. 2 (Pt. 2) (April 2002): S1–93, cited on the National Center for Biotechnology Information Web site, http://www.ncbi.nlm.nih .gov/pubmed/12180494.

Gregory Gordon:

167   Gregory Gordon, "NutraSweet: Questions Swirl," posted at Gregory Gordon, United Press International Investigation, http://www.dorway.com/ upipaper.txt, accessed August 5, 2008.

"helped get Searle's petition":

169   Ibid.

"four more FDA officials":

169   Ibid.

"a financial bonanza":

171   Ibid.

Asda, for example:

173   Jess Halliday, "Asda Reformulates to Cut Out Artificial Additives," *Food and Drink Europe, Decision News Media,* May 18, 2007, http:// www.foodanddrinkeurope.com/news/ng.asp?n=76642-asda-additives-private-label, accessed August 5, 2008.

"has pledged":

174   Ibid.

"[U.K. Wal-Mart] will also meet":

174   Ibid.

"consumer awareness of nutrition":

174   Ibid.

Coca-Cola Great Britain:

175   Food and Drink Federation, "Hot Issues: Additives: Information on Spe-
       cific Companies," http://www.fdf.org.uk/hot_issue_additives.aspx#item9,
       accessed August 5, 2008.

The country's most popular soft drinks, Coke and Diet Coke, have
never contained these colours, and recent launches such as
Schweppes Straightcut sparkling drinks contain no artificial colours or
flavours.

We continually evolve our products across our range to meet the
needs of British consumers and we do recognise the changing tastes
and interest in product ingredients, including additives. This is why
we changed Fanta Orange earlier this year, removing the artificial
colours it contained.

All ingredients in our products are clearly labelled on pack and
more information can be found via *www.coca-cola.co.uk* or by calling
the freephone Consumer Careline on 0800 227711.

on May 27, 2008:

175   Laura Crowley, "Sodium Benzoate Removed from Diet Coke," *Food
       Navigator—Europe,* May 27, 2008, http://www.foodnavigator.com/
       Financial-Industry/Sodium-benzoate-removed-from-Diet-Coke, accessed
       August 6, 2008.

Kraft Foods U.K.:

175   Food and Drink Federation, "Hot Issues: Additives."

We continue to study information regarding ingredients and food
additives, as well as follow recommendations of regulatory agencies on
this issue. Where appropriate, we take these findings into considera-
tion as part of our ongoing review of product formulations and reformulation efforts. . . .

Our products are clearly labelled. Consumers in the UK seeking
further information about our product ingredients can contact our
consumer careline: 0800 783 7106.

See also www.krafthealthyliving.co.uk.

Mars U.K.:

175   Ibid.

The first focus has been our biggest-selling brands and in November 2007 Starburst Chews became free from all artificial colours. Packs now carry a logo to show there are 'no artificial colours and flavours'.

In December 2007, Skittles were made free from all the artificial colours highlighted in a landmark study by Southampton University, commissioned by the Food Standards Agency. We have already removed four colours mentioned in the Southampton study from Peanut and Choco M&M's, and are in the process of removing the final one so they too will be free from these artificials during 2008. Our work to remove artificial colours is continuing and we are actively reviewing the use of additives across our whole brand portfolio. If they are used, additives are clearly listed on the packs to inform consumers.

See also marsconsumercare.co.uk.

Nestlé U.K.:

175   Ibid.

In 2005, Nestlé Rowntree was one of the first major confectionery manufacturers to commit to using no artificial colours in its sweet ranges, such as Fruit Pastilles, Jelly Tots, Frooty Tooties and Fruit Gums. Recent confectionery reformulations include: Smarties moving to a new 'no artificial colours' recipe in 2006; in June 2007, the level of real fruit juice in Rowntree's Fruit Pastilles, Fruit Gums and Jelly Tots was raised to 25%; and from September 2007, the UK's favourite kids' chocolate brand—Milky Bar—is to be made with all natural ingredients.

See also www.nestlé.co.uk.

U.K. Cadbury Chocolate division:

176   Ibid.

This programme has been underway for over a year, starting with Bassett's Allsorts and Jelly Babies. On top, we recently launched a new range of products, which is free of artificial colours, under the brand name of The Natural Confectionery Company. We will replace all artificial colours in the rest of our sweets during 2008.

See also www.cadbury.co.uk/en/ctb2003.

"Explaining its decision":

176   BBC News, "Asda to Cut Out Additives by 2008," May 15, 2007, http://news.bbc.co.uk/2/hi/business/6657757.stm, accessed August 6, 2008.

"Reformulation was hard work":

176   "Healthy Eating, Food Additives, Feel Good with Asda," Wal-Mart U.K. Web site, http://www.asda-feelgood.co.uk/healthy-eating/food-additives, accessed August 6, 2008.

Chapter 7. The Ring of Fire

Kennedy's book:

184   Robert F. Kennedy, Jr., *Crimes Against Nature* (Harper Collins, 2004).

the price of food:

186   Economic and Financial Indicators, *The Economist* commodity-price index, *The Economist*, June 2008.

prescriptions for our children:

186   *Generation Rx: A Film* by Kevin P. Miller, Common Radius Films, Vancouver, B.C., 2008, http://www.generationrxfilm.com/home.html.

quite a hefty sum:

191   University of California Newsroom, "UC, Monsanto reach $100 million settlement in growth hormone patent case," February 27, 2006, http://www.universityofcalifornia.edu/news/article/10237, accessed August 6, 2008.

BIO 2008:

191   Alan McHughen is a University of California, Riverside, CE plant biologist in the College of Natural and Agricultural Sciences Botany and

Plant Sciences, http://www.facultydirectory.ucr.edu/cgi-bin/pub/public
_individual.pl?faculty=1912, accessed August 6, 2008.

Dr. McHughen has suggested:
191 Alan McHughen, *Pandora's Picnic Basket: The Potential and Hazards of
Genetically Modified Foods* (Oxford University Press, 2000).

"Most of us have":
191 Revolution Health, "Healthy Living, The Real Problem with Genetically
Modified Foods," *Alternative Medicine Magazine,* December 13, 2006,
http://www.revolutionhealth.com/healthy-living/natural-health/health
-food-store/health-hazards/genetically-modified-food, accessed August 6,
2008.

"computers in the university's":
192 Susan Benson, Mark Arax, and Rachel Burstein, "A Growing Concern,"
Mother Jones, January/February 1997, http://www.motherjones.com/news/
feature/1997/01/biotech.html, accessed August 6, 2008.

"the pope of food allergies":
193 Marcia Garcia-Lloret, MD, Director of Food Allergy Clinic, Mattel Children's Hospital, University of California, Los Angeles, personal communication, October 2007.

FDA on additives:
193 Center for Science in the Public Interest, *Integrity in Science Database,*
as cited: "Hugh A. Sampson, "Study Concerning Effect of Aspartame on
Headache Received Funding from NutraSweet," *New England Journal
of Medicine* 317 (1987): 1181–85; "Has Received Research Support from
Pharmacia-Upjohn," *New England Journal of Medicine* 346 (2002):
1294–98. "Member, Generally Recognized as Safe (GRAS) Expert Panel
on Behalf of DMV International for the Use of Bovine Lactoferrin as a
Food Ingredient. (Notification to FDA, GRAS Notice No. GRN 000077,
5/2/01)," accessed August 6, 2008.

U.S. Patent and Trademark Office:
143 U.S. Patent 7381556, Nucleic acids encoding deallergenized proteins and
permuteins. Inventors: Murtaza F. Alibhai, James D. Astwood, Charles A.
McWherter, Hugh A. Sampson. Assignee: Monsanto Technology, LLC.

Issued by the United States Patent and Trademark Office, June 3, 2008. Patent Storm, http://www.patentstorm.us/patents/7381556.html, accessed July 8, 2008.

A. Wesley Burks, MD:

194 See BiomedExperts, the first literature-based scientific social network, Research Profile on Wesley Burks, http://www.biomedexperts.com/Profile.aspx?n=A_Wesley_Burks&auid=173748, accessed August 7, 2008.

peanut allergy vaccine:

194 Food Allergy Hope, "Making Sense of Science," ScienCentral News, March 17, 2005, http://www.sciencentral.com/articles/view.php3?language=english&type=&article_id=218392504, accessed August 7, 2008.

"Dr. Burks has reported":

194 Y. M. Donald et al., for the TNX-901 Peanut Allergy Study Group, "Effect of Anti-IgE Therapy in Patients with Peanut Allergy," *New England Journal of Medicine* 348, no. 11 (March 13, 2003): 986–93, http://content.nejm.org/cgi/content/full/348/11/986, accessed August 7, 2008.

"has consulting arrangements with":

194 Scott H. Sicherer and A. Wesley Burks, "Maternal and Infant Diets for Prevention of Allergic Diseases: Understanding Menu Changes," *Journal of Allergy and Clinical Immunology* 122, no. 1, (July 2008): 29–33; published online June 11, 2008, http://www.jacionline.org/article/S0091-6749(08)00955-X/abstract, accessed August 7, 2008.

food allergy articles:

195 Dennis Clements, Connect with Your Health Care at Duke Medicine, Advice from Doctors, Food Allergies, http://www.dukehealth.org/Health Library/AdviceFromDoctors/YourChildsHealth/food_allergies: "Individualized treatment plans should be prepared in advance and medications readily available. These medications may include antihistamines (Benadryl, for example) and injectable epinephrine (EpiPen)." Accessed August 29, 2008.

"play God":

198 Michael Pollan, "Playing God in the Garden," *New York Times,* October 25, 1998, http://query.nytimes.com/gst/fullpage.html?res=9D03EFD

8143DF936A15753C1A96E958260&sec=&spon=&partner=permalink &exprod=permalink, accessed August 7, 2008.

"genetic roulette":

198 Jeffrey M. Smith, *Genetic Roulette, The Documented Health Risks of Genetically Engineered Foods* (Yes! Books, 2007).

Britain's Advertising Standards Authority:

199 Linus Gregoriadis, "Monsanto GM Food Ads Found to Mislead, Four Complaints to Watchdog Upheld, While Nine Are Rejected," *The Guardian*, August 11, 1999, http://www.guardian.co.uk/news/1999/aug/ 11/food.foodanddrink. Cited on the blog North Coast Voices, "Naughty Naughty Monsanto," August 25, 2008, http://northcoastvoices.blogspot .com/2008/08/naughty-naughty-monsanto.html.

Philadelphia jury:

199 Ken Dilanian, "Philadelphia Jury Rules Against Monsanto in Chemical Contamination Case," *Philadelphia Inquirer*, August 24, 2000, http:// www.accessmylibrary.com/coms2/summary_0286-6488815_ITM. Cited on the blog North Coast Voices, "Naughty Naughty Monsanto."

Alabama jury:

199 Michael Grunwald, "Monsanto Held Liable for PCB Dumping," *Washington Post*, February 23, 2002, p. A01, http://www.washington post.com/ac2/wp-dyn/A54914-2002Feb22?language=printer. Cited on the blog North Coast Voices, "Naughty Naughty Monsanto."

In December 2007:

200 Trevor Wells, "Monsanto Busted for Contempt of Advertising Authority in South Africa," Mathaba News Network, December 23, 2007, http://www.mathaba.net/0_index.shtml?x=575597. Cited on the blog North Coast Voices, "Naughty Naughty Monsanto."

"available scientific data":

201 Bong S. Sarmiento, "Diocese on Bt Corn: Vatican Compendium Cites 'Precautionary Principle,' " *MindaNews*, February 1, 2005, http://www .organicconsumers.org/ge/vatican20705.cfm, accessed August 7, 2008.

sued Monsanto:

202 Personal communication with Michael K. Hansen, PhD, senior staff scientist, Consumers Union, conducted on May 29, 2008.

"yield may even decrease":

202 J. Fernandez-Cornejo and M. Caswell, "The First Decade of Genetically Engineered Crops in the United States," USDA Economic Research Service, http://www.ers.usda.gov/publications/EIB11, accessed August 7, 2008.

reduced *yields:*

203 Food and Agriculture Organization, "The State of World Food and Agriculture 2004. Biotechnology: Meeting the Needs of the Poor?" http://www.fao.org/newsroom/en/focus/2004/41655.

A 2007 study:

203 B. Gordon, "Manganese Nutrition of Glyphosate-resistant and Conventional Soybeans," *Better Crops* 91, no. 4 (2007): 12–13.

"in the United States":

203 M. Qaim and D. Zilberman, "Yield Effects of Genetically Modified Crops in Developing Countries," *Science* 299 (February 7, 2003): 900.

The USDA has just waived:

204 Garance Burke, "USDA Axes National Survey Charting Pesticide Use," *Boston Globe,* May 22, 2008, http://www.boston.com/news/nation/articles/2008/05/22/usda_axes_national_survey_charting_pesticide_use, accessed August 7, 2008.

May 2008 Vanity Fair:

204 Donald L. Barlett and James B. Steele, "Investigation: Monsanto's Harvest of Fear," *Vanity Fair,* May 2008, http://www.vanityfair.com/politics/features/2008/05/monsanto200805.

Monsanto just highlighted:

205 "Strong Results in Roundup, Seeds and Traits Businesses Propel Monsanto to Record Third-Quarter and Year-to-Date Results," News Release, Monsanto Corporation, http://monsanto.mediaroom.com/index.php?s=43&item=619, accessed August 7, 2008.

In order to ensure:

205   "For the Record, Is Monsanto Going to Develop or Sell 'Terminator' Seeds?," Monsanto Corporation, News and Media, http://monsanto .mediaroom.com/index.php?s=59&item=136?s=59&item=136, accessed August 7, 2008; "Our Products: Leading Brands," Monsanto Corporation, http://www.monsanto.com/products/brands.asp, accessed August 7, 2008.

Another cost to farmers:

205   "Monsanto Announces Indemnity Collection System for Unauthorized Bollgard Cotton Grown in Brazil," Monsanto Corporation, News and Media, March 20, 2006, http://monsanto.mediaroom.com/index.php?s =43&item=369&printable?s=43&item=369&printable, accessed August 7, 2008.

GM seeds typically cost:

205   Soil Association, "Seeds of Doubt: Experiences of North American Farmers of Genetically Modified Crops," http://www.soilassociation.org/seeds ofdoubt; Soil Association, "GM Crops Are Economic Disaster Shows New Report," June 5, 2003, http://www.soilassociation.org/web/sa/ saweb.nsf/librarytitles/GMO12092002.html, accessed August 7, 2008.

"herbicide-tolerant" crops:

205   Ibid.

the safety of GM foods:

207   Jeffrey M. Smith, *Seeds of Deception, Exposing Government Lies About the Safety of the Genetically Engineered Foods You're Eating* (Yes! Books, 2003), p. 7.

"We are assured that":

208   Ibid., p. 15.

The press went wild:

208   Ibid.

Former president:

209   BBC News, "1999: Scientists Highlight Hazards of GM Food," February 12, 2003. H. A. Kuiper et al., "Adequacy of Methods for Testing

the Safety of Genetically Modified Foods," *The Lancet* 354 (1999): 1315–16.

"the British food industry":
209   Smith, *Seeds of Deception,* p. 26.

British Medical Association:
209   Ibid., p. 30. Marie Woolf, "People Distrust Government on GM Foods," *Sunday Independent* (London), May 23, 1999.

the European Parliament:
209   USDA Foreign Agricultural Service, Global Agriculture Information Network, "Russian Federation Biotechnology Federal Law Sets Biotech Labeling Threshold at 0.9 Percent," October 30, 2007, http://www.fas.usda.gov/gainfiles/200711/146292887.doc; Smith, *Seeds of Deception,* p. 30.

Monsanto found itself:
210   ETC Group, "Monsanto Monopoly Patent Under Scrutiny," News Release, April 28, 2003, http://www.purefood.org/patent/monsanto050103.cfm, accessed August 7, 2008.

Dr. Florence Wambugu:
210   Corporate Watch, "Corporate Critical Research: Microsoft: Gates Gets Wambugu-ed," http://www.corporatewatch.org.uk/?lid=364, accessed August 7, 2008.

Dr. Wambugu's critics:
210   Lim Li Ching, "Broken Promises," December 5, 2004, http://www.i-sis.org.uk/BrokenPromises.php?printing=yes, accessed August 7, 2008; "Throwing Caution to the Wind," a review of the European Food Safety Authority and its work on genetically modified foods and crops by Friends of the Earth, Europe, November 2004, http://www.foeeurope.org/GMOs/publications/EFSAreport.pdf; Lobby Watch, http://www.lobbywatch.org/profile1.asp?PrId=131, accessed August 7, 2008.

In June 2003:
210   BBC News, "Blair's Legal Reforms Under Fire," June 14, 2003, http://news.bbc.co.uk/2/low/uk_news/politics/2989672.stm, accessed August 7, 2008.

"The only human GM trial":

210 Andrew Osborn, "Brussels Clears GM Maize to Please US," *The Guardian,* January 29, 2004, http://www.guardian.co.uk/world/2004/jan/29/usa.foodanddrink, accessed August 7, 2008.

News articles:

210 Ibid.; BBC News World Edition, "Meacher Attacks GM crops," February 18, 2003, http://news.bbc.co.uk/2/hi/uk_news/politics/2771129.stm, accessed August 7, 2008.

the biotech industry:

211 Toni Johnson, "Sprouting EU Feed Wars," November 20, 2007, http://www.cfr.org/publication/14840/sprouting_eu_food_wars.html, accessed August 7, 2008; EuropaBio, the European Biotechnology Lobbying Group, "Biotech Crop by Country," http://www.europabio.org/documents/200501/ISAA%20backgrounder.pdf, accessed August 7, 2008.

GM corn:

211 Ibid.

In October 1999:

211 Stanley W. B. Ewen and Arpad Pusztai, "Effect of Diets Containing Genetically Modified Potatoes Expressing Galanthus Nivalis Lectin on Rat Small Intestine," *The Lancet,* 354 (October 16, 1999), http://www.bioemit.math.ntnu.no/meetings/pusztailancet.pdf, accessed August 7, 2008.

"The situation is like":

211 Smith, *Seeds of Deception,* p. 44.

"I've been reviewing":

212 World Intellectual Property Organization, Patent Applications: WO2005/015989 and WO2005/017204, http://www.wipo.int/portal/index.html.en; "Monsanto Files Patent for New Invention: The Pig, Greenpeace Researcher Uncovers Chilling Patent Plans," August 2, 2005, Geneva, Switzerland, http://www.greenpeace.org/international/news/monsanto-pig-patent-111, accessed August 7, 2008; "No Patents on Seeds, The Pig Monopoly (Monsanto)," http://www.no-patents-on-seeds.org/index.php?option=com_content&task=view&id=29&Itemid=20.

Myriad Genetics:

213 Teresa Riordan, "Dispute Arises Over Patent for a Gene," *New York Times,* October 30, 1994, http://query.nytimes.com/gst/fullpage.html?res =9D06EEDB113FF933A05753C1A962958260, accessed August 7, 2008; Teresa Riordan, "A Dark Horse Has Scored a Victory in the Race to Commercialize a Gene Linked to Breast Cancer," *New York Times,* August 18, 1997, http://query.nytimes.com/gst/fullpage.html?res=9806E5 DC113FF93BA2575BC0A961958260, accessed August 7, 2008.

600,000 U.S. women:

213 Riordan, "Dispute Arises Over Patent for a Gene."

"Mr. Wyden had put":

214 Ibid.

"Women gave their blood":

214 Ibid.

Myriad Genetics' patent:

214 Philippa Brice, "Myriad Loses BRCA1 Patent Appeal," October 22, 2007, http://www.phgfoundation.org/news/3854, accessed August 7, 2008; "Myriad Genetics Awarded Three U.S. Patents and Eight International Patents," May 15, 2001, http://www.myriad.com/news/release/210288, accessed August 7, 2008.

Chapter 8. This Is a Carrot

Christopher Robin to Winnie the Pooh:

268 A. A. Milne, *The House at Pooh Corner* (Dutton Juvenile, 1988).

Appendix: Organic 101

A recent study:

271 David Derbyshire, "Organic food really IS better for you, claims study," *The Daily Mail,* October 28, 2007, http://www.dailymail.co.uk/news/ article-490255/Organic-food-really-IS-better-claims-study.html#

eating organic food:

271   "Study Hails Organic Foods Benefits," *BBC,* October 29, 2007, http://
      news.bbc.co.uk/1/hi/england/tyne/7067226.stm, Carlo Leifert, "Quality
      Low Input Food" study, Newcastle University, Quality Low Input Food,
      http://www.qlif.org, Biological Farmers of Australia Co-op Ltd. March
      27, 2007, http://www.bfa.com.au/_files/20070327_Organic%20IS%20
      Healthier.pdf, Maria L. Amodio, Giancarlo Colelli, Janine K. Hasey,
      Adel A. Kader, "A comparative study of composition and postharvest per-
      formance of organically and conventionally grown kiwifruits," University
      of California Davis, *Journal of the Science of Food and Agriculture,* as pub-
      lished in *Chemical and Industry* magazine on March 26, 2007,
      p 1228–1236, DOI: 10.1002/jsfa.2820

Organic food also had:

271   The Times Online, "Official: organic really is better", *The Sunday Times,*
      October 28, 2007, http://www.timesonline.co.uk/tol/news/uk/health/
      article2753446.ece

Additionally, according to:

272   The Center for Food Safety, *Genetically Engineered Food,* http://www
      .centerforfoodsafety.org/geneticall7.cfm, accessed June 2008.

Made with Organic:

272   United States Department of Agriculture, Agricultural Marketing Pro-
      gram, National Organic Program, Organic Labeling and Market-
      ing Information, http:www.ams.usda.gov/AMSv1.0/getfile?dDocName
      =STELDEV3004446&acct=nopgeninfo, United States Department
      of Agriculture, Agricultural Marketing Program, National Organic Pro-
      gram, Regulation by Part, Labeling Preamble, http://www.ams.usda.gov/
      AMSv1.0/getfile?dDocName=STEKDEV3003509&acct=noprule
      making

no established guidelines:

274   United States Department of Agriculture, Agricultural Marketing Pro-
      gram, National Organic Program, Organic Labeling and Marketing In-
      formation, http://www.ams.usda.gov/AMSv1.0/getfile?dDocName=STEL

DEV3004446&acct=nopgeninfo, Debbie Safarti and Nell Behnfield, Whole Nourishment, Nourishing News, August 2007, http://www.whole nourishment.com

According to the Environmental Working Group:
274 Food News from the Environmental Working Group, *Get the Guide: The Full List: 43 Fruits and Veggies,* http://www.foodnews.org/walletguide.php

INDEX